Food, Feelings & Freedom

Learn How to Manage Your Emotions and Take Control of Your Eating in 8 Weeks

G.G.CLEMENT

First published by Ultimate World Publishing 2024
Copyright © 2024 Gina G Clement

ISBN

Paperback: 978-1-923255-05-0
Ebook: 978-1-923255-06-7

Cover design: Ultimate World Publishing
Layout and typesetting: Ultimate World Publishing
Editor: James Salmon

Ultimate World Publishing
Diamond Creek,
Victoria Australia 3089
www.writeabook.com.au

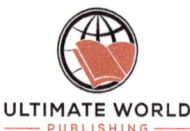

Disclaimer

This book contains information for educational and informational purposes only. It is not intended as a substitute for individual professional psychological, dietetic, or medical advice. Readers are encouraged to consult with qualified professionals in these fields regarding their specific situations and circumstances.

Pseudonyms are used for all individuals mentioned in this book to ensure their privacy. These stories are composite illustrations reflecting common experiences with emotional eating. Any resemblance to actual persons, living or deceased, is purely coincidental.

This book's strategies, techniques, and recommendations are based on professional expertise, research, and anecdotal experiences. Results may vary, and success is not guaranteed, as it depends on the reader. The author and publisher disclaim any liability for the decisions made by readers based on the information presented in this book.

Readers should also be aware that the emotional and psychological content is not a replacement for intensive therapy or counselling. If you are experiencing mental health concerns, it is recommended that you seek support from registered or licensed mental health professionals.

For those who want to change their now,
believe in yourself and make it happen…

Contents

Introduction

You've probably heard of emotional eating, even if it's not something you've personally dealt with. When I told people I was writing a book about changing emotional eating behaviour, they showed excitement. However, their enthusiasm waned when I mentioned the key component was managing emotions. This book and subsequent program aren't a quick fix or a magic pill, so they might not be everyone's cup of tea. But for those ready to take charge of their eating habits, they're here to help.

This book is divided into four parts, each serving a different purpose. The first two chapters lay the groundwork, setting the stage for understanding emotional eating and its impact on our lives. They delve into the reasons behind emotional eating, touching on the roles of our emotions, external influences, and personal experiences. The focus here is self-awareness, recognising emotional triggers, and discovering alternative ways to cope without turning to food.

Chapters 3 to 6 introduce the program's core elements: food, activities, and mindset. These sections provide practical strategies to tackle emotional eating head-on. You'll learn to see food as fuel, shift your perspectives, develop meal-planning skills, and follow guidelines. Activities become an interim crutch, and you'll dive into the significance of self-care.

Chapters 7 to 10 of the book dive into practical strategies for progress monitoring, goal-setting, overcoming obstacles, and knowing when it's time to conclude the program. These sections guide you through the process of tracking your journey, setting achievable goals, and navigating challenges along the way. Emphasising self-awareness and reflection, these chapters equip you with tools to identify triggers, adjust strategies as needed, and recognise when you've reached your desired outcomes. You'll explore effective goal-setting techniques, strategies to stay motivated, and the importance of celebrating achievements. Additionally, these chapters offer insights on recognising when you've achieved your goals and how to gracefully transition out of the program when the time is right.

Finally, chapters 11 and 12 reveal the heart of the program. We'll combine all the elements and resources and outline how they work together to support your journey towards conscious eating habits and emotional literacy.

1

Let's Get Started

Have you often heard or believed that you turn to food when emotions run high? In a world where emotional eating is the norm, often unspoken and unnoticed, have you detected a pattern within your own experiences or those of your family? Food and drink intertwine with every facet of our lives, acting as a source of solace or celebration, whether the occasion is joyous or sad. In many societies, the inclusion of food and drinks in social gatherings is customary. It is a cherished tradition that, in moderation, can be embraced with open arms. Yet one must tread cautiously, for the hazards of emotional eating will manifest differently for everyone, casting doubt and uncertainty upon its presence in our lives.

Emotional eating is the most commonly known eating behaviour in the world. It emerged as an identified eating pattern back in the 1980s through eating behaviour questionnaires. Other patterns, such as external and restrained eating, were identified, but they're less well known than emotional eating.

Originally, emotional eating was defined as eating in response to negative emotions. But it has evolved and now includes eating due to positive and neutral feelings, which makes sense. Eating as a reaction to emotions can really mess with your eating habits and weight management goals, and can physically lead to extra kilograms, stubborn weight loss, and even binge-eating episodes. It is not something you want at all.

Emotional eating doesn't just mess with you physically; it also has some sneaky mental side effects. Guilt is an unwelcome guest that shows up unannounced after you've had a little too much indulgence. And, if you allow it, it can lead you down a dark path to feeling down or depressed. Unbeknownst to you, emotional eating can mess with how you feel about and see yourself and throw a wrench into your relationships with others.

Do you fit the emotional eater bill? Let's put your self-awareness to the test - take a moment to think about these questions:

- When life throws you for a loop, you're stressed, or everything becomes too much, do you seek comfort in food?

- If you're feeling down, sad, happy or excited, do you eat more than the usual amount of your favourite foods?
- Do you think about or eat food when you're happy or want to reward yourself?
- If you overeat or eat the wrong food while on a diet, do you instantly give up and eat whatever you want for the rest of that meal or for that day?
- Do you find yourself eating food without being hungry or having a reason to eat it?

If you instinctively say *Yes,* or *Mostly Yes,* in response to these questions, it's time to accept that you may be an emotional eater. Is this revelation new to you, or have you suspected there is a powerful link between your feelings and eating habits?

Eating behaviour can be broken down into two key components. First, we have a connection between our emotions and eating habits. Next, we have the level of control we wield over the food and drinks we consume. Visualise these components as two spectrums, one representing the interplay between our emotions and food choices, and the second highlighting our power to regulate what we eat.

Reaching for chocolate when you're feeling highly emotional is an example of the emotion–food connection. Whether you eat one row or the whole family block indicates your level of control over what you eat.

Take a look at the diagram below. Can you find your spot on each spectrum? For emotional eaters, you might climb high on the emotion spectrum, where feelings call the shots, while reactive eaters may find themselves on the lower end of the control spectrum, where food and influence take control. People who are not emotional eaters but have no control over what they eat can overeat due to external cues. If pinpointing your current position feels like a tough task, don't worry. You can always revisit this question once you've gained more insights into your relationship with food and your capacity for food control.

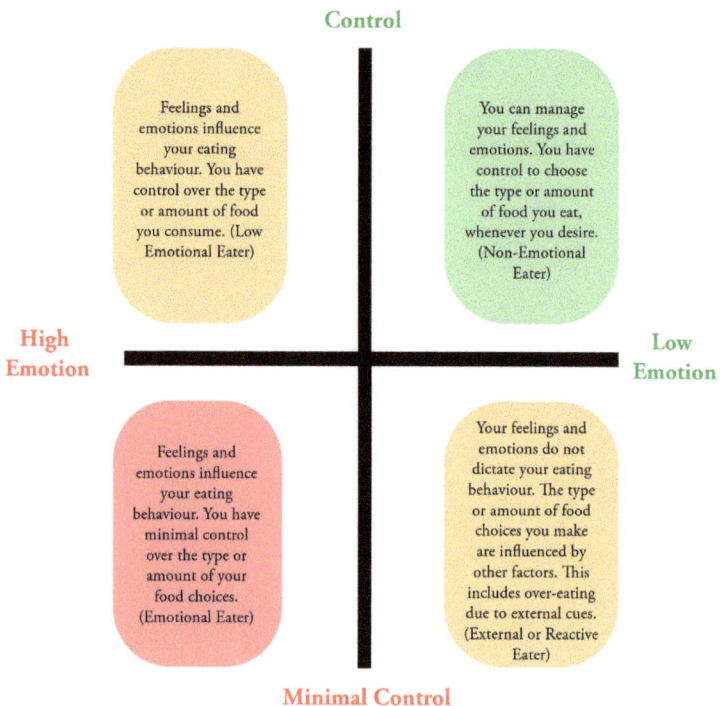

Control

Feelings and emotions influence your eating behaviour. You have control over the type or amount of food you consume. (Low Emotional Eater)

You can manage your feelings and emotions. You have control to choose the type or amount of food you eat, whenever you desire. (Non-Emotional Eater)

High Emotion

Low Emotion

Feelings and emotions influence your eating behaviour. You have minimal control over the type or amount of your food choices. (Emotional Eater)

Your feelings and emotions do not dictate your eating behaviour. The type or amount of food choices you make are influenced by other factors. This includes over-eating due to external cues. (External or Reactive Eater)

Minimal Control

Emotion vs Control

Does your position on the diagram truly resonate with you, or do you feel one of the other quadrants might be a better fit? Are you content with your current position, or do you want to be in a different quadrant? If the latter, which specific quadrant would you prefer, and what motivates this desire for something different?

Let's delve more into how emotional eating can impact your life. Is it hindering your progress or preventing you from achieving certain goals? One common response to this question relates to the struggle to shed kilograms and maintain weight loss. You enthusiastically start a new meal plan, cruising smoothly through the initial days or even the first couple of weeks. But then, something happens that throws you off balance, stirring up emotions. Do you keep on track, sticking to your meal plan while ignoring the emotional whirlwind? Or does your will break, and you seek solace in comforting foods to help you cope?

Unmanaged emotional eating can wreak havoc on various aspects of your life, especially your physical health. Losing weight turns into an uphill battle when you find yourself caught in the never-ending tug-of-war between staying true to your *current diet* and surrendering to those emotional triggers lurking around every corner. This can lead to considering extreme measures to control weight such as weight loss injections and bariatric surgery. And even if you decide to go for bariatric surgery, which alters the size of or bypasses your stomach, there's no guarantee it will transform you into a lighter, healthier version of yourself. The cold truth is that bariatric surgery solely tackles the quantity of food you consume, not the magical transformation of your food choices into healthy options. That responsibility falls squarely on your shoulders.

Post-surgery, emotional eaters still grapple with the impact of their emotions because surgery can't fix that part. True success with bariatric surgery requires managing emotional eating before the procedure and learning about healthy eating habits. It's an holistic approach that goes beyond the operating room.

Emotional eating is a sneaky habit that creeps up on us when our emotions run wild. Food or drink becomes our trusty sidekick, ready to rescue us from the depths of our feelings. Speaking of habits, they often get a bad rap. We associate them with things we need to change or get rid of. But habits can also be *positive*, and we often don't realise it. Take a moment to think about activities like walking the dog, staying hydrated, or making our bed. These little habits bring some extra goodness into our lives, and we slip into them effortlessly without even thinking twice.

As an aside, did you notice how I use the word *positive* instead of *good*? It's a subtle shift but an important one. By using the word p*ositive,* it implies a direction of moving forward, without passing judgment. Therefore, we're not judging whether the habit is inherently *good* or *bad*.

So, back to talking about habits. The tricky thing about emotional eating as a habit is that the longer you wait to tackle it head-on, the tougher it becomes to manage and change. These eating patterns have been etched into your life, resistant to change, but it is possible to forge new positive habits.

Eating habits don't impact only you; they ripple out into the lives of those around you, especially children. If you happen to be a parent or guardian, those curious eyes watch your every move. Children are like little copycats, unknowingly imitating your actions and learning your emotional eating habits. Take a moment and think how often you have dished up their favourite snacks as rewards for their victories, or handed them treats to ease their sorrows after being sad or losing at something. It happens more often than you realise, and before you know it, you've unintentionally taught them to rely on food and drinks to navigate their emotions.

Emotional eating can also significantly impact your finances. You might not have given it much thought, but those impulsive food choices driven by your emotions can wreak havoc on your budget. Have you ever found yourself going way overboard, spending more than you had planned on your weekly food purchases?

But how does it happen, you wonder? Imagine a scenario where something's troubling you, and instead of sticking to the dinner meal you had planned at home, you give in to the temptation of ordering that mouthwatering pizza. Or perhaps you're feeling utterly bored at work, and out of nowhere, you decide to visit the nearby café, splurging on fancy coffee and cake instead of nibbling on the humble muesli bar you brought from home. And let's not forget those times when frustration, anger, or sadness hit you during a shopping trip. Suddenly, your cart is filled with all those irresistible extras: biscuits, chocolate, or snacks. Items that are way outside the boundaries of your well-intentioned shopping list. Before you know it, those impulsive purchases start adding up, leaving you with a hefty bill week after week. Do you know the true financial cost of your emotional eating?

When we're talking about food, we can't overlook the cost of wasted food, which hits your wallet and takes a toll on the environment. Think about all those instances when your emotions led you astray at mealtimes, causing you to toss out unused fruit, vegetables, or meat you had every intention of using, but that expired before you could use them. What about when you were feeling disappointed and only managed to finish three-quarters of that extra-large meal you ordered? The last thing on your mind was the impact on your wallet or the environment as you dumped the remnants in the rubbish.

If these consequences of emotional eating resonate with you, or you have reasons for wanting to gain control over it, there is hope - you have the power to make a positive change. Many individuals have successfully overcome emotional eating, and

I'm here to guide you on that journey, too. The solution we will explore in the upcoming chapters is refreshingly simple. It builds upon existing knowledge and harnesses the power of psychology to empower you to make lasting changes. As an additional bonus, the psychological concepts we'll delve into can be applied to other emotional issues.

By now, you might be intrigued by the program but still harbour doubts about its effectiveness. The fact that you've picked up this book and made it almost through the first chapter suggests that you possess a glimmer of hope and a willingness to be convinced. Let me present it to you this way: you've realised that emotional eating is taking a toll on your life and possibly affecting the lives of those around you. However, the fear of embarking on another failed diet or food program lingers in your mind. What lies ahead is different from a traditional diet as this isn't a diet at all. It's about acquiring the tools and knowledge to effectively manage your emotions when it comes to eating. This program offers you the freedom to choose what you eat, whether you prefer to cook at home, purchase from a store, or explore the options provided by a weight management service. The power is firmly in your hands. If your ultimate goal is weight management, you can progress to that once you have mastered your emotional eating patterns.

Let's confront another concern that may be nagging at you: the fear of failure. Failure doesn't exist in this program. Instead, I want you to change your perspective and see every task as an opportunity to practise and grow. Think back to when you were learning to walk. Did you master it on your very first attempt? Unlikely! You probably stumbled or fell and persevered until you could walk confidently without a second thought. Every skill you've ever acquired—whether it's walking, talking, reading, riding a bicycle, driving a car, drawing, playing an instrument, building a house, or even flying a plane—requires practice. Failure wasn't a stumbling block but rather a stepping stone on the path to success. By shifting your mindset and embracing failure as an opportunity to practise and improve, you open yourself up to limitless possibilities.

If you're about to embark on this incredible journey of managing your emotions and reclaiming control over your relationship with food, having a support system in place can make all the difference. Many of you, especially women, tend to believe that you must bear the weight of the world on your own, never daring to ask for help and constantly putting the needs of others before your own. Some of you may think you must show you're strong and capable, not vulnerable and needing help. These mindsets can be your downfall. To give yourself the best chance at success, it's time to embrace a little bit of selfishness, prioritise your own well-being, and find your very own cheer squad.

Research has shown that having a supportive network significantly boosts motivation and increases the odds of achieving success. Whether it's finding a trusty buddy who's by your side, joining a program, becoming part of an inspiring group, or connecting with an encouraging online community, having that strong support system in place will keep your motivation firing and drive you toward your goals. Not only will you receive an abundance of encouragement and positive vibes along the way, but you'll also have someone to hold you accountable and provide that extra push when you need it most.

It is possible to undertake this program without external support. It's a journey that demands self-motivation and unwavering determination. However, you all will encounter those moments when your motivation wanes and the temptation to throw in the towel becomes all too enticing. That's precisely where a support system swoops in to save the day. It helps you overcome doubts, stay on track, and reignite your determination.

Are you ready to tackle your emotional eating? Let me ask it another way. Are you ready to commit at least 80% effort to follow the program to tackle emotional eating? "*What is 80%?*" you ask. If you are confident that you can achieve what you set out to do without second-guessing your decision, that is what I refer to as 80%. If the answer is "*No, not yet*", then the time isn't right and that's absolutely fine. Please keep doing what you're doing. I genuinely appreciate your dedication to learning about emotional eating. When the moment feels right, you can always come back and pick up where you left off.

If you don't think you can commit to 80% effort, hold off and return to this book when you feel more prepared. This threshold is crucial for ensuring your success. Don't be hard on yourself if you decide to wait until you can fully dedicate yourself to this journey. It simply means you're being mindful of your own readiness and ensuring that you embark on this adventure with the right mindset.

However, if you're raring to go and ready to give at least 80% effort, then you're ready to dive into the next chapter and embark on this transformative adventure.

2

A Relationship
with Food

Before you can start changing things, knowing what you're dealing with and what you want to achieve is important. This is about re-writing your life as you presently know it. Have you noticed that once you've mastered something, it becomes second nature, like riding a bike? This also goes for our thoughts, feelings, and reactions. Much of it is based on what we've learned, and we keep rolling with it, often without even realising it. To break free from this autopilot mode, we've got to hit the pause button and become aware of what's happening inside our minds. It's like shining a spotlight on your thoughts, how you connect with others, and the situations you find yourself in.

Now, on the topic of eating, it's also something we do without really thinking. Have you ever found yourself munching in front of the TV without even noticing, only realising your plate is empty when the show ends? Or having a good time with friends and not paying attention to how much you eat or drink? And those moments when you're snacking because you're bored – it's like the snacks vanish before you know it. This all happens without us really noticing, and that's where the magic of awareness comes in. To make changes, to learn, to take charge – you've got to be in the know about what's going on and your role in it.

Awareness is the first step in steering your thoughts, emotions, and actions in the right direction. As an added bonus, the power of awareness extends far beyond just changing your eating habits – it's an insight that can be used in other areas of your life.

Let's dive into your eating behaviour. Have you ever wondered what really shapes how you eat? If you're someone who follows their hunger cues and picks foods that align with what your body needs, kudos to you. You're one of the *minority*, and this book might not interest you. Notice how I put extra weight on the word *minority* here. For the majority of people, eating isn't just about listening to their hunger. It's determined by schedules, trendy diets, TV ads, or even catching a whiff of something delicious as they stroll by. Their menu depends on what's around, how much time they've got, what's convenient and budget-friendly, and how they're feeling at the moment. Rarely does it boil down to whether that food is truly the right kind of fuel for their bodies at that point.

Let's return to that Emotion vs Control diagram we talked about earlier. Can you see yourself fitting into one of those sections, or are you still puzzling it out? In the upcoming sections, we'll dig into how these two aspects shape your eating habits and what that means for you. When it comes to the *Emotion* spectrum, the real game-changer is becoming aware of your emotions and getting to know them. Believe it or not, this might be the trickiest part of the program. It involves recognising and putting a name to feelings like sadness, anxiety, frustration, excitement, or boredom. Only then can we delve into how these emotions tie into your eating habits – the when and the what? If you're not exactly sure about what you're feeling and can't quite put a finger on it, don't worry. It's okay to hit pause on reading and take a moment to explore your feelings. Because even if you can't put a name to an emotion, you can still sense its presence in your body.

Have you ever experienced any of these bodily sensations?

- Feeling queasy or those fluttery butterflies in your stomach
- A parched mouth that has you swallowing more often than usual
- Finding yourself a little extra sweaty
- Palms getting a bit clammy

- The irresistible urge to fidget, shift, or even tremble
- Your heart is beating faster, and/or your breathing is shallower and quicker

These sensations can signal different things – nervousness, anxiety, excitement, or fear. What they mean depends on the situation that triggers them. Imagine someone getting ready for a first date, facing an impending exam, gearing up for a speech in front of a crowd, or getting set to compete in a sports event – all these experiences could bring about those sensations.

Have you experienced any physical sensations, especially if you're feeling sad or helpless?

- A squeezing sensation in your chest
- A weighty feeling in your stomach and limbs
- A prickling sensation in your throat
- Maybe your eyes even welled up a bit

Let's shift gears and explore a different side of things. How about experiencing:

- A sense of lightness in your chest
- Limbs and body that feel loose and relaxed
- A mind that is crystal clear
- A surge of energy that gets you motivated to do things
- For no apparent reason, an urge to break into a smile

I'm willing to bet you've realised these could be the physical manifestations of joy, satisfaction, pride, or other positive and uplifting emotions. Paying attention to how your body reacts is the key to unlocking how you learn and understand your feelings.

The Control spectrum involves being able to manage your food choices consciously. For some, being in command of what they eat comes naturally, while for others, the sway of suggestions and influences can be quite impactful. The food and beverage marketing wizards know this vulnerability inside out and tailor their campaigns to trigger these suggestive impulses. Have you ever wondered what to have for dinner, and the recent delicious-looking pizza ads prompt your mind to consider that a realistic option? It's like that age-old wisdom – never shop when you're hungry. You toss more delicious treats into your cart than you initially planned, especially lured in by the aroma of food courts and anything else that catches your senses.

True control means having a firm grip on your choices and the confidence to stand by your decisions. This mainly affects those who react externally rather than those who turn to food for emotional comfort. While some emotional eaters manage to keep a strong hold on their food urges, others might find themselves swayed by emotions and a lack of restraint. If you've recognised that suggestions tend to shake up your food choices, have you pinpointed what your weaknesses are? Is there a particular food that's your kryptonite – the one you can't resist? No matter how resolute your intentions are, whenever that situation arises, you surrender to the pressure, only to feel guilt afterwards. That guilt can snowball, leading you to consume more than you intended, making you even more frustrated with yourself. Does this sound familiar to you?

Society and expectations from family and friends also affect our eating behaviour. Celebratory feasts have existed forever, whether in medieval times, via biblical references or for family gatherings. Celebrations are special events that occur infrequently and are a time of socialising, excitement and recognising a momentous occasion. Socialising with friends and family also involves consuming food and drink, which can be challenging to manage when it occurs frequently. Socialising is very important as we need a sense of connection with others for our well-being. Some people, however, may find enjoying the company of people is being overshadowed by the importance and desire for food and drink.

So far, we've spoken about your role in your eating behaviours, but not the role that food fulfils. We know food is an energy source and a tool required for existence, so how can it have a role? For something to have a role, it has to be given meaning, value and expectations, similar to what we include in any other relationship. We're not talking about a person here; we're talking about food! People place more meaning and value on a tool or inanimate object they appreciate. You may be familiar with other tools around the house: a lawnmower in the garden shed, a pen to write with, a fork to eat with, or anything we engage with. If we extend this list of tools further to include other tools used to live our lives, do you consider them to have the same practical value as the abovementioned lawnmower or pen? The car or bicycle you use for transport, the money you have, the clothing you wear, the smartphone you use, and the food you eat? With some tools, we give them a higher value and status than they literally have, therefore fulfilling a role that we give them. With emotional eating, the value placed on food elevates it, similar to the role of being a *best friend* to a person, in that it consoles, celebrates, distracts, is a confidante, companion or buddy, and at times fights against you.

To gain control and not be emotional eaters, we need to de-throne food from being the *best friend* and consider it a tool required for life. This can only be done if you are ready to acknowledge that this could be how you view food and are prepared to change how you engage with it. You may go through a period of sadness and uncertainty where you feel a sense of loss. This is the same as experiencing grief, as you're choosing to distance yourself from something that was meaningful and valued. It's okay to feel like you're not ready to make this change in your life, as it's a big step to turn away from or break up with something that has helped get you through good and bad times. If you're not ready yet, take some time to understand the role you give to food, as well as what foods you choose to eat and when you choose to eat them. This awakening may take some time because you may not want to confront the reality that you use food to handle your emotions. Also, you may feel scared that if you take the food away, your feelings are laid bare and then what do you do…

Millions of dollars are spent annually on mental health and weight management programs or products. Still, the anxiety, depression and weight of people in developed countries continue to increase … Why?

If you ever find yourself at the crossroads of wanting to change, but *you're* resisting because *you* need to put some effort in, say to *yourself* the following:

> "If I do *nothing*, I stay the same. Regardless of what I read, *nothing* will change from where I am right here, right now."

Or,

> "If I do *something* towards helping myself, and it doesn't matter how insignificant or small that is, at least I'm doing *something*."

What are your immediate thoughts after reading these? Are you a *nothing* or a *something*? If you're leaning towards *nothing*, that's okay. Have a breather, gather your thoughts, and when you're ready to do *something*, this book will be here to guide you. If you're prepared to do *something*, keep reading and understand that every step you take towards what you want to achieve, counts.

These are some of the key steps in exploring your relationship with food:

- Being aware of your emotions
- Understand what food means to you
- What needs to happen before you can change your behaviour

We've established that awareness is the first essential step in behavioural change. This applies to any behavioural change: becoming a better driver and mastering reverse parking; getting over a fear of water and learning to swim; realising that your fear of being judged is hindering your work prospects; understanding your controlling behaviour might be due to feeling anxious or discovering that your dependence on food is used to cope with your emotions. The simplest explanation of being aware is to exist in the present, here and now, and use our thoughts and bodily senses to focus on what we want to be aware of.

Let me introduce you to Lexa and Casper, whom you will see becoming aware of how they used food to cope with their emotions.

Lexa is a 40-something-year-old with two high school teenagers and works part-time as a dental surgery receptionist. Lexa's partner works full-time and has a stressful job, so the house and family responsibilities often fall upon her. Lexa's demands at work have increased, and she finds it challenging to juggle work, children and home responsibilities. If work has been busy, she'll call into the convenience store to buy chocolate or a pastry to give herself a 'lift' and help cope with the rest of the day. When busy with the family after school, she'll often be too tired to prepare a meal, so she relents and gives in when the family suggests ordering a takeaway. If work or the family has been stressful, her 'go-to' is sitting in front of the television food channel with a couple of glasses of wine and savoury crackers. She has put on weight since her last child and feels uncomfortable with her body, but she doesn't have the motivation to do anything about it; she can't bear to look at herself in the mirror, and instead of doing something about changing the situation, she looks for comfort and support in her favourite foods.

Lexa became aware of her relationship with food by working through some examples of her daily activities and considering any behaviour patterns involving food. Why did she need the after-work chocolate bar? Why give in to the family and order takeaway food? Why drink wine or resort to eating comfort foods? Often, food decisions were made around feelings, be it tiredness, frustration, stress, guilt, or low self-esteem. Subconsciously, Lexa knew she was using food like this, and she felt ashamed to admit she relied on food to help her get through her days. She agreed to monitor her emotions daily for a week with the reassurance that she could learn to manage her feelings better and stop using food as a crutch. Fortunately, Lexa knew her feelings and could name them when they occurred. Lexa wrote in the *Food & Feelings Diary* for a week; by then, she could see the patterns emerge where she used food to cope with or manage her feelings. She was encouraged to take note of her mind and body sensations and practise naming her feelings whenever possible. This didn't take away her discomfort at times, but it is relevant to managing emotional eating and life. Below is an excerpt from her *Food & Feelings Diary*.

Food & Feelings Diary

Day and Time Tuesday	Place	Food/Drink	Was this on your plan?	Mood before	Mood after
10:30	Work	Double shot latte Chocolate muffin	-	Tired, stressed	More energy, can face the day
12:30	Work	Chicken and salad	-	Wanted a break from work	More energy and enjoyed the meal
4:45	Petrol station	KitKat and Pepsi Max	-	Tired and going home to a busy family	Guilty!
6:30	Home	Spaghetti bolognese and gelato	-	Relieved I had something to heat up	Could sit, relax and watch TV with son

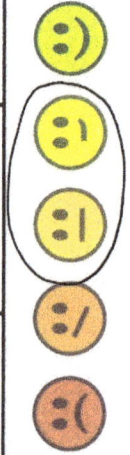

Overall, my day was: (circle)

26

The next step is to examine the food you consume and why you make those choices. If you started using the *Food & Feelings Diary*, can you notice any patterns in the food choices? What about the meaning, value or expectations you place on your chosen food?

- *She craved something sweet and enjoyable after a day at work as she was tired from being around people all day and frustrated that she couldn't relax due to family and household needs. She wanted the 'treat' to give her a burst of energy and a few moments of enjoyment before facing the busyness of home.*
- *She noticed that when she is too tired to cook at home, she is easily persuaded to order takeaway despite knowing the food may not be healthy. In this situation, the food is being used to appease the family, and it is less effort for her as she doesn't have to cook or clean up.*
- *If she has had a stressful, tiring or challenging day, she looks forward to her favourite activity of escaping in the food channel on television, and drinking a couple of glasses of wine with whatever snacks she has in the pantry. She sees this as her 'me' time, and the role of the wine and snacks is to use alcohol as a form of enjoyable relaxation with the snacks as an accessory.*
- *She knows she should do something about her increasing weight and discomfort but doesn't have the energy or motivation to make a start and put in the effort to succeed. This is when she uses her favourite 'pick-me-up' foods to have a brief respite from feeling bad about*

herself. She knows this doesn't help her long-term, but she is looking for a short-term 'fix'.

When Lexa realised what she was using food for, she became sad and embarrassed. She was using food and alcohol to cope with how she was feeling, and in some cases, it provided a brief respite from experiences in her day-to-day life.

Casper is a 28-year-old person who lives alone in a rented apartment. They are a full-time accountant in a small accounting firm. Casper recently graduated, so they are trying to increase their experience and confidence at work. Often this means they work longer hours than they're being paid for. Work for Casper is stressful, and they're frustrated that tasks take longer than they do for the other experienced workers. On stressful days they use the routine drive home to think about a nice meal that will help them feel better. More often than not, their decided meal will be home delivery as they're too exhausted to cook. Casper has a small group of friends with whom they socialise occasionally. They prefer to keep to themself, either reading, gaming or watching movies. They don't mind being around people, but they're nervous about meeting and talking to people whom they meet socially. When they socialise with their friends, Casper usually has 3 to 4 quick alcoholic drinks to give them confidence and reduce their nervousness when talking to strangers.

Casper became aware of their relationship with food and alcohol by working through some examples of their days and considering any behaviour patterns involving what they consumed. Why did they need to focus on treating themself after a stressful or exhausting day at work? Why drink alcohol to cope with being sociable? Casper wrote in the *Food & Feelings Diary* for a week; by then, they could see the patterns emerge where they used food to cope with or manage their feelings. They didn't realise the extent of using food to help cope with work-related feelings. Unlike Lexa, Casper wasn't fully aware of their feelings. They knew they needed alcoholic drinks to cope with social occasions. Still, they weren't aware why, so Casper was encouraged to take note of their mind and body sensations and practice naming their feelings whenever possible. Below is an excerpt from their *Food & Feelings Diary*.

Food & Feelings Diary

Day and Time	Place	Food/Drink	Was this on your plan?	Mood before	Mood after
THURSDAY 7³⁰	HOME	JUST RIGHT & COFFEE	–	TIRED & NOT HUNGRY	SATISFIED I ATE SOMETHING
10¹⁵	WORK	ENERGY DRINK MUESLI BAR	–	STRESSED	MORE ENERGY & GUILTY
12⁰⁰	WORK & HJ'S	DBLE WHOPPER COMBO	–	NEEDED SOMETHING TO PICK ME UP	BETTER & GUILTY.
4²⁰	WORK	FROZ LASAGNE & COKE	–	STRESSED, TIRED FRUSTRATED HAVE TO WORK LATE	ENERGY TO KEEP GOING

Overall, my day was: (circle)

30

To understand how you view the food you choose, ask yourself the following questions:

1. What did you choose to eat?
2. Why did you choose it?
3. What did you hope to achieve by making this choice?

Be brutally truthful when answering questions 2 and 3, as it's easy to answer this how you think you *should* respond instead of revealing the ugly truth. If you're struggling to answer question 2 as to why you chose what you did, compare it to something else and see if that prompts some ideas. For example, why did you decide to eat biscuits instead of an apple, as both are equally available? They are both accessible, though biscuits are more convenient to eat as they take less effort than eating an apple. What about how you value the biscuits versus the apple? The biscuits are a *treat*, and you anticipate they will taste enjoyable to eat, whereas the apple is a healthy choice and *good for you*, but it doesn't trigger the same anticipation as the biscuits.

Often, you don't know what you hope to achieve when eating some foods because you eat unconsciously. Increasing awareness about your use of food can be uncomfortable and something you may not want to admit, as it puts the spotlight on your feelings. Did you choose the biscuits because you're bored and wanted something *nice* to do for a couple of minutes? The same applies to using them as a distraction if you procrastinate and want to stall doing something. Or, you finally completed a task and wanted a small reward to celebrate. If you can't identify why you chose the biscuits, it could be a long-established habit with no reason except that you routinely do it. Any or none of these may resonate with you, but hopefully you get the idea that sometimes you must explore your feelings and actions a bit more deeply than you're used to.

Once you realise why you make the food choices you do and are ready to admit that you use food and beverage choices to help manage your emotions, you want to do something about it, but you're not sure you have what it takes to succeed. You may not realise it, but questioning your food choice and becoming aware has already changed what you know about yourself and how you view the food you eat. Sure, you might slip up and eat unconsciously, but this is the beginning of increasing awareness and gaining control. The *FoodFeelingsFreedom* program has been designed to build on your current understanding and desire to change your behaviours without requiring much willpower from yourself. If you need more time to think about your situation, then take the time necessary, as every day you will become aware of your emotions, and thinking about the food you eat is better than if you did nothing at all.

Frequently Asked Questions:

Q. What if I don't understand why I eat?

A. If you still don't understand why you choose the food you do, despite asking yourself the three questions above, you can still follow the program and gather insight as your behaviour changes. If you don't want to proceed until you understand, talk to a friend, a coach, or a health professional to help you dig deeper into your behaviours.

Q. What if I don't think I have a relationship with food?

A. If the food you choose does not relate to how you feel at that time, and you have reasonable control over what and why you eat, then you are probably correct. Maybe pass on this book to someone you know who struggles with emotional eating.

Q. What if I'm scared to admit that I can't manage my emotions without using food?

A. That is a normal response, and it's okay to be uncertain about how you will cope with your emotions. If it's too much to consider now, you can start when you're ready. In the meantime, you can take some little steps by being aware of your feelings and food choices. The program is designed to help you change your behaviours without feeling like you've lost your previous support. If you don't think you can do this yourself, find a supportive buddy or a coach to support you.

Something to think about

- Use the *Food & Feelings Diary* daily for a week to understand what and why you choose to eat or drink something.

- Think about your expectations of consuming food and beverages.

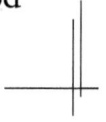

3

The Three Elements

Changing your behaviour can be really tough, especially when it's a habit you've had for a long time. This program was designed to make the process of changing your eating behaviour easier whilst also improving your emotional awareness and self-management skills. The program consists of three elements that are valuable on their own, but when combined, they can help you achieve even greater results. Although you may have tried one or all of these elements before, using them together in this specific order and for this particular purpose can truly transform your approach to eating.

Here are the three essential elements of this program:

1. Food – Includes Meal Planning and using Food as Fuel: This is about making thoughtful choices about

what you eat and recognising that food nourishes your body.

2. Engaging in Activities: Incorporating activities into your routine can help distract from emotional eating and promote a healthier and richer lifestyle.

3. Managing Your Mindset and Emotions: Understanding and managing your emotions is crucial. By doing so, you'll be better equipped to make positive changes in your behaviour.

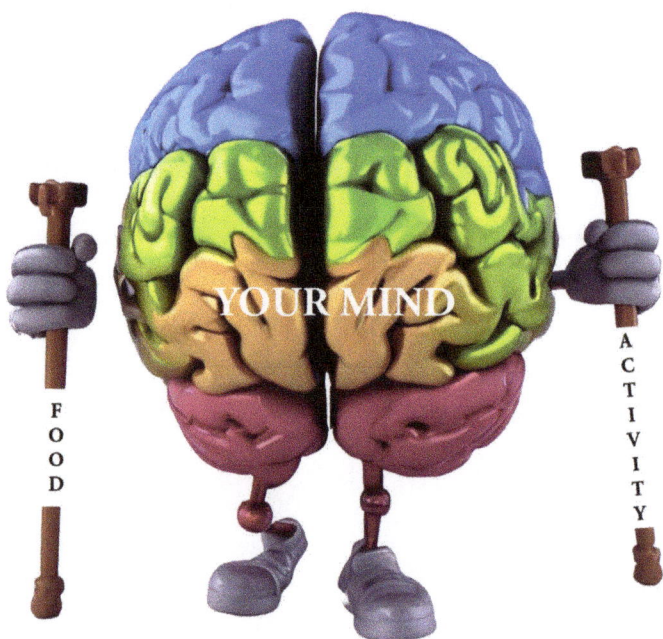

YOUR MIND

F
O
O
D

A
C
T
I
V
I
T
Y

The Three Elements

Food as Fuel

This section focuses on changing how you see food and reducing the emotions tied to it. The goal is to loosen your strong emotional connection with food, which is essential for overcoming emotional eating. As mentioned earlier, we often attach significant value to certain everyday tools. In this case, we're talking about the food we purchase and consume. When you decide to buy an ingredient or a meal, what factors come to mind? Do you think about the nutritional components, the brand, societal perceptions, or how it will make you feel when you eat it?

At its core, food is a tool—a source of nutritional energy that fuels our bodies and sustains life. Everything beyond this basic function is a value we assign to it. This program will reintroduce the idea of thinking about food solely as an energy source without the added emotions and value judgments clouding your perspective.

To help you grasp this concept better, let's consider how we view friendships. Think about your *best friend* or someone you highly value as a friend. What sets them apart from your regular friends? You likely share more emotional experiences with them; they've been there for you during joyous and challenging times. In contrast, a *regular friend* with whom you don't share such a deep emotional connection is more neutral. Have you ever had a falling-out or become distanced from your best friend, causing you distress as you lost a valued and important support system?

Now, let's apply this analogy to food. Consider food as you would your best friend. Think about how important it is to you, how it supports you through good and bad days, and how it's always there, perhaps even more consistently than your *real* (human) best friend. Our goal is to lessen your emotional ties with food and relegate it to the status of a regular friend. While this comparison may seem unusual, take some time to reflect on whether it resonates with you.

If you believe this process will be daunting or painful, don't worry. You don't have to navigate it alone. This book will provide you with strategies to minimise the emotional distress associated with this transition. This includes reshaping your perception of food and planning your meals every two weeks. Meal planning is a widely used technique for managing food behaviours, but in this program, it serves as a behavioural activity that reduces emotion, particularly anticipation and worry surrounding eating and food choices.

Activities

The second step in this program involves making a conscious choice to engage in activities instead of resorting to food as a way to handle your emotions. These activities can be anything that suits your schedule and budget. You're absolutely right to think that we're essentially substituting food with something else to manage your emotions. This is a transitional phase where you use alternative activities, like a temporary crutch, while you learn to manage your emotions without relying on food. This intermediate step is crucial because it makes your emotions more manageable to handle without falling back into the old pattern of using food as a crutch. It's your opportunity to get accustomed to a new version of yourself where food no longer dominates your attention and disrupts your life.

These activities don't have to be grand or complicated; they can be as simple as spending 15 minutes outdoors in the sunshine. Here are some examples: reading a chapter from a book, going for a 20-minute walk, listening to music for 30 minutes, playing with a pet for 15 minutes, browsing social media for 30 minutes, engaging in a hobby for 30 minutes, or anything else that piques your interest. If you're struggling to come up with ideas, you can refer to the extensive list in Chapter 12 and choose activities from there.

You'll have a general list of activities, with some specifically designated for certain situations, such as for reward or feeling-boosting moments. Remember that the goal is to replace previous food-related choices with engaging in an activity. Besides being beneficial in the long run, there are built-in safeguards to prevent you from developing any unfavourable habits related to the frequency of these activities.

These safeguards are in the form of Activity rules. Here is an example of an Activity rule and why it's important.

Rule: You can engage in a particular activity a maximum of two times per week.

Explanation: Restricting how often we do an activity helps us maintain our interest, enjoyment, and enthusiasm. It might seem counterintuitive because we often think that doing something more frequently leads to greater interest and enjoyment. Isn't this why we binge-watch entire series, play video games for hours, or devour a packet of chocolate biscuits in one go? However, this isn't the case. In reality, our brain chemicals work in the opposite direction here. When we repeat the same activity too often, we don't look forward to it as much because we know it's happening regularly; our excitement diminishes, and eventually, we lose interest. The novelty wears off, and we start craving something new. Limiting each activity to a maximum of two times per week can prolong the enjoyment and enthusiasm you derive from it. This approach prevents you from rapidly cycling through your list of activities and reduces the risk of becoming overly reliant on one specific activity.

Mindset

The third aspect of this program involves managing your thoughts and emotions without relying on crutches like food, shopping, alcohol or anything else. Even if you've made progress with meal planning and shifted your activities away from food-centric choices, you've only tackled the physical aspects of emotional eating, which is the halfway point. At this stage, you may have gained more awareness and some control over your emotional eating, and it might feel like you've conquered it. But remember, you're still leaning on a crutch and haven't completely mastered your emotions.

This is where the final part comes into play—learning to manage your emotions. It's the *superpower* of the three elements because its effects are not immediately visible; it influences the other two components and is essential for achieving lasting success.

Many people discover it's simpler and more comfortable to take physical action to aid themselves rather than tackling the mental task of managing their emotions and mindset. Therefore, you might be tempted to take shortcuts and skip certain elements—after all, who wouldn't want to bypass the tedious and challenging aspects and get straight to the goal? However, in this case, if you skip any of these three components, there are no guarantees that you'll ultimately overcome emotional eating. These elements are interdependent; omitting one or two may yield short-term or partial success, but in the long run, you'll likely find yourself right back where you started—a bit like a behavioural boomerang.

This is how you can explore the key elements:

- Transforming Your Relationship with Food: We'll explore how to shift your perspective on food.
- Effective Meal Planning: Discover the art of planning your meals for success.
- Swapping Food for Activities: Learn how to replace food with engaging activities.
- Mastering Your Emotions and Mind: Find strategies to gain control over your emotions and mindset.

Understanding Food: Description vs. Evaluation

How often do you take a moment to see food as merely a source of nutritional energy? Chances are, not very often unless you are an elite athlete or a dedicated bodybuilder. For most of us, food doesn't appear in our minds as it is. Instead, we tend to focus on how it influences our emotions, whether it's good or bad for our health or whether it adheres to societal norms.

One effective way to shift your perspective on food is to describe it in its purest form. This involves conducting a literal inventory of the food item, utilising your body's senses of sight, hearing, smell, taste, and touch to paint a vivid picture of it. Some of these ideas might ring a bell if you've ever engaged in a mindfulness exercise centred around food. If this concept is new to you, let me introduce you to Casper's experience.

For this exercise, Casper selected an apple. Initially, when I asked Casper to describe what they saw, their response was rather vague: *"A smallish red apple"*. I encouraged them to be more specific and literal in their observations. Here's what Casper provided after my prompt:

> *"It's mostly round with some bumps at the bottom. The apple exhibits various shades of red, with some green patches at the lower end. There's a pale brown stalk emerging from the indentation at the top. There's a green sticker on one side with the brand name in white letters."* With this more detailed description, Casper was on the right track. We then proceeded to the sense of hearing, but it didn't yield much information. Casper tapped on the apple and described the sound as "dull and soft, consistent all around the apple." Next, we explored the sense of smell, but Casper couldn't detect any particular scent from the apple. Moving on to the sense of touch, Casper shared, "It's mostly firm, with some softer spots. The surface feels smooth all over, except for the stalk area, which is woody and rough. The bumps encircle the indentation at the bottom." We saved the sense of taste for last, allowing Casper to take a bite of the apple. Before biting into it, I prompted Casper to pay attention to the experience. Here's what Casper conveyed about the bite:

> *"The apple felt firm against my teeth. I needed to exert some effort to pierce the skin, and I heard a satisfying crunch as I bit into it. The piece inside my mouth had*

a chunky texture, maintaining its firmness against my teeth and tongue. I could taste and smell a delightful blend of sweet and tangy flavours released from its juices."

When asked to examine the bite mark their teeth left on the apple, Casper noted, "There are clear teeth marks at the top of the bite. You can distinguish the reddish skin from the creamy inner flesh. And, if I smell the apple now, I can detect a subtle, crisp sweetness." This exercise helped Casper truly engage with their sensory experience of the apple, enhancing their awareness and connection to the food they were about to eat.

I can assure you that after a few rounds of describing food or drinks in this manner, your perspective on them will shift significantly. You can apply this exercise to anything you consume, whether it's a piece of fruit, a biscuit, a chocolate bar, or even your meal tonight.

Another method to alter your perception of food is by breaking it down into its macronutrients, which include protein, fats, and carbohydrates. This can be a bit challenging for foods that lack ingredient labels; you'll need to refer to a food ingredient list or use a suitable app to gather this information. Every food item contains varying amounts of these macronutrients, as illustrated in the list below.

Food	Protein (g)	Carbohydrate (g)	Fat (g)
Apple, medium	1	25	0
Hard cheese, cheddar 100g	25	4	35
Chocolate, milk 100g	8	60	30
Cream, heavy 100ml	2	3.1	35
Crisps, salted 100g	7	50	38
Egg, hard-boiled 100g	13	1	11

Source: Fatsecret calorie counter app

Examining a food's macronutrients is the ultimate way to describe it based on its nutritional energy source. However, this approach may seem quite intense unless you're working toward a specific goal. If you find this idea intriguing, you can explore it further through your local gym, consult a dietitian, or search for information online.

These sensory experiences and macronutrient breakdowns are two approaches to reshaping how you perceive food, reducing its emotional charge and perceived value. I hope you can see that you have the power to view food differently than you do currently. Without even realising it, you've grown accustomed to using emotionally charged or judgmental words when thinking about and describing food. I understand that this might sound a bit confusing at first, so let me clarify with an example from Casper.

In my initial conversation with Casper about describing food, I asked them to share how they would describe some of the regular foods they typically consumed. Here's what Casper had to say about their morning muesli: "*Healthy, crunchy, and good for me*". Out of these words, only "*crunchy*" truly described a characteristic of the muesli. "*Healthy*" and "*good for me*" were possible evaluations of the muesli. Regarding chocolate biscuits, Casper used words like "*milk chocolate, smooth, melty, crispy, and naughty*". While some of these words had a bit of description, "*naughty*" clearly represents an evaluation of the chocolate biscuit. When describing ice cream, Casper used the words "*creamy thickness, cold, white and orange in colour, icy, decadent, and fattening*". Right away, you can see that some words describe the ice cream's attributes, while others place a value judgment on the product—either from a personal or societal perspective. We can detach ourselves from the emotions typically associated with these foods by steering clear of value-loaded words when describing our food. This helps us view them more literally and objectively.

Meal Planning

Earlier in the chapter, I mentioned how meal planning is a behavioural activity that helps dial down the emotional rollercoaster surrounding your food choices. Have you ever realised how much time and mental energy you devote to planning your meals? Perhaps you think about what you'll eat the following day while lying in bed at night. Or do you start thinking about dinner options right after finishing lunch? Do you obsess over what dinner might lift your spirits on dull or gloomy days, spending the whole day in meal contemplation or planning? These behaviours keep food at the forefront of your mind and intensify its importance and emotional connection.

Creating a meal plan for a fortnight (two weeks) in advance offers your mind some much-needed freedom to focus on other aspects of life during this time and takes the spotlight off food. We all need to eat and share meals socially, but if we're to break the emotional grip that food holds over us, we must consciously and noticeably shift our behaviour. Remember that everyone's meal plan will vary depending on family dynamics, work commitments, available time, freezer space, and preferences, and it could change from one fortnight to the next.

In the following chapter, we'll explore the details of how to design your two-week meal plan. There are specific rules governing meal choices that are crucial in the early stages of the program, and these rules will relax as you gain control over your relationship with food. The pace at which you loosen these rules will depend on your individual progress, as everyone navigates these stages differently. If you find that loosening the rules results in losing control over your relationship with food, you can always revert to following them again.

Eating out and socialising around food are common activities in our lives. These can still be accommodated within your two-week meal plan but with a change in perspective.

The primary focus will shift from fixating on the food to engaging in meaningful conversations and enjoying the company of friends, family, or colleagues. A specific rule will be introduced for dining out, allowing you to participate in social gatherings while reducing the emphasis on food.

The stages of meal planning:

1. Pre-program Preparation (Week Zero)
   - Decide on your meals for the upcoming two weeks.
   - Determine if you'll prepare, purchase in advance, or make meals as needed.
   - Keep a record of your meal choices for the coming fortnight.

2. Fortnightly Meal Plan
   - Stick to the meal plan you've outlined.
   - Adhere to the established rules.
   - Note any thoughts, feelings, or self-discoveries during this period.
   - Record any adjustments to your food choices for the following fortnight.

3. Preparation for the Next Fortnight
   - This step takes place in the second week of each fortnight.
   - Document and prepare your meal plan for the next two weeks.

4. Repeat Stages 2 and 3
- Continue cycling through stages 2 and 3 until you successfully complete the program
- Continue to follow the rules and relax them when suggested.

Below is Lexa's meal plan for the first fortnight and some of the challenges she had to consider.

Lexa recognised the importance of accommodating her own needs and those of her children and partner to ensure the success of her two-week meal plan. Knowing that the evening meal held the most significance for her family, she made it the centrepiece of her plan, implementing meal restrictions mainly for breakfast and lunch. She initiated a discussion with her family, explaining her intention to plan their evening meals for the next two weeks and the reasoning behind it. Lexa didn't feel the need to consult the family regarding breakfast, lunch, or snack options since everyone made their own choices for those meals. In addition to gathering meal suggestions from her family, Lexa considered their availability and time constraints when preparing meals. Given their busy schedules, particularly with numerous after-school activities and limited weekday cooking time, Lexa found incorporating ready-made or store-bought meals into their Monday-to-Friday routine practical. To streamline the process, Lexa and her teenagers pre-cooked and froze some meals, reducing the week's cooking workload and alleviating her anxiety. They also stocked up on bulk takeaway meals, providing convenience for the family. Lexa had a standing lunch appointment with colleagues each Wednesday at the same café; she was happy to have the same menu selection every week.

Fortnight Meal Plan 🍓

Flexible meal choices

Spaghetti bolognese (x2)

Beef stroganoff + pasta (x2)

Baked salmon + veges (x2)

Steak + veges

Sausages + veges

Sweet + Sour Pork + rice

Lasagne + veges + chips

Nachos

Chicken cashew stir-fry + rice

Pizza (supreme, pepperoni)

Roast chicken + veges

_____

_____

_____

Breakfast ☐ Lunch ☐ Dinner ☐
1. Toast (Jam, vegemite)
2. Eggs Benedict
3. Weetbix and banana
4. Muesli and blueberries

Breakfast ☐ Lunch ☐ Dinner ☐
1. Chicken and salad
2. Ham salad sandwich
3. Salmon and asian salad
4. Donor Kebab and chips

Snacks and Desserts
1. Double chot latté
2. Honey greek yoghurt
3. Red wine
4. Gelato

Eating Out

Cafe/restaurant and menu choice
Oriental Pearl • Sweet + Sour Pork and rice ; red wine
Jimmy's Yeeros • Donor kebab and chips
Royal café • Ham salad sandwich and Latté

Swapping Food for Activities

To make the switch from using food as an emotional crutch to engaging in alternative activities, it's essential to maintain a written list of activities you can turn to when you're feeling emotional. While you might consider keeping a mental list, it's not the most practical approach as it can be challenging to remember and keep track of. Here's a step-by-step guide:

1. Begin with a Clean Slate: Start with a blank page or use the *Activity List* worksheet available on the *www. FoodFeelingsFreedom.com.au* website.
2. Listing Activities: Add activities you either already engage in or want to try. Keep in mind the essential rules, which we'll discuss shortly. If you're unsure about what activities to include, consult the comprehensive list provided in Chapter 12.
3. Prioritise Feeling and Mood Boosters: Start by listing specific activities that have the power to lift your mood or serve as rewards. These are critical because they are the primary reasons for seeking solace in food. Ensure that the rewarding activities provide you with a similar sense of satisfaction as your previous food rewards. The same principle applies to activities that serve as pick-me-ups; opt for ones that genuinely elevate your mood. Begin by listing at least four activities for each of these categories. If you've relied on food for dealing with specific emotional triggers, add activities specifically tailored to address those triggers.

4. Combatting Boredom: Remember that boredom is a feeling often overlooked. If you find yourself mindlessly scavenging the fridge or pantry out of sheer boredom, be sure to include activities explicitly designed to counter this sensation.

5. General Activity List: Once you've addressed specific emotional areas, move on to create a list of general activities that can be used at any time. Initially, aim to have between six to ten activities on this list. Don't be daunted by the quantity; remember the rules. You cannot repeat the same activity more than twice per week. Include familiar activities, but also add some you're interested in trying. Be creative and imaginative. This list is not a daily to-do list you must complete; it's a collection of potential activities you can draw from throughout the week. This is especially important to note for those who are accustomed to daily must-do lists and experience anxiety when they are not completed. If this describes you, refer to the specific section in Chapter 5 that addresses managing this mindset.

It's crucial to understand that if you're choosing an activity for reasons like exercise, work, study commitments, health concerns, or any other goal unrelated to the primary objective of diminishing your preoccupation with food, you should follow those specific requirements without adhering to the program's Activity rules.

<u>Here are some key points to keep in mind:</u>

Exercise or Movement: Ensure you engage in exercise or physical activity daily for your health and fitness routine. The rules do not restrict this.

Work or Study: Carry out your work or study tasks as required or to meet deadlines. The rules do not apply in these situations.

Here is Lexa's list of activities. She began by prioritising her "reward" and "when stressed" activities, focusing on listing them first. When it came to brainstorming general activities, she initially struggled because she couldn't envision herself engaging in even two or three, let alone ten, in a week. I encouraged her to compile at least six, emphasising that they should be realistic and genuinely pique her interest, regardless of whether she'd get to do them or not.

Activity List

Do a jigsaw puzzle

Watch youtube

Read a novel

Learn to draw

Have a bubble bath

Watch television

Read a magazine

Do some stretching

Spring clean a room

To reward myself

Watch the Food channel

Phone a friend

Have a mini massage

Play an online game

When I am ... stressed !
At work — go outside for 5-10 mins
— walk around the block
At home — listen to calming music
— do some gardening

To comfort myself
Sit somewhere quiet

Sit in the garden + look at the plants

Spend time with the dog

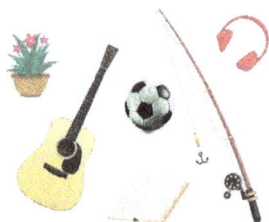

Other ...

Mastering Your Emotions and Mind

This element of the program focuses on psychological challenges. Here, you'll embark on a journey to understand, experience, and manage your emotions in a healthy way. Starting from week three, we introduce you to the program's mental and intangible aspects. Just like acquiring any new physical or mental skill, you'll need to dedicate time and effort to practising the weekly tasks until they become second nature. Once you've acquired and integrated these skills, they'll become valuable tools you can use throughout your life, ready to be deployed whenever you confront emotional challenges. That's why we refer to this element as the *Superpower*.

Throughout the program, we'll explore the following topics:

- Emotional awareness
- Acknowledge and identify bodily sensations
- Describe emotions
- Choose to embrace emotions
- Take control

As Lexa embarked on the psychological aspect of the program, she experienced a mixture of excitement and anxiety. She understood that this was the heart of the program, the reason for her commitment, but she was apprehensive about confronting her emotions. Having relied on emotional eating for many years, she harboured doubts about transforming her behaviour in just eight weeks. Nevertheless, after only two weeks of diligently following the meal planning and food-to-activity substitution strategies, she noticed a reduced emotional dependence on food. This motivated her to commit to the weekly exercises, and she vowed to practice them extensively. Lexa recognised that the initial stages might be challenging, but she believed that consistent practice was the key to replacing her former unhealthy habits. Her progress was not without its setbacks. It often felt like she took two steps forward and one step back. Despite the occasional sluggish and tricky progress, Lexa's confidence grew with each passing week. When weeks five and six approached, she needed more time to practice confronting her emotional challenges. Consequently, she opted to repeat these weeks, and took the opportunity to relax some of the food and activity rules. This extension allowed her to reinforce her newfound skills. Lexa felt assured she could maintain her newly acquired abilities when she commenced the final stage of reframing her thoughts. She eagerly anticipated the transformation in her approach to managing her emotions. To her surprise, she discovered that these skills were not confined to the program's context; they seamlessly transferred to other aspects of her life. Moreover, she observed that her family indirectly benefited from her newfound strategies.

This program's psychological guidance and instructions are intended for general purposes and should not be considered a substitute for specialised or personalised psychological treatment. If you are presently undergoing counselling or receiving support from a mental health professional, you are advised to consult with them regarding the appropriate timing for engaging with the psychological content and exercises. Your mental health professional can offer insights and guidance tailored to your specific needs and circumstances.

Frequently Asked Questions:

Q. What if I struggle to stick to my meal plan?
A. Don't lose heart. If you find it challenging to adhere to your meal plan, don't despair. There are underlying reasons that might affect your ability to stay on track. Your task is to identify these obstacles and understand what's impeding your progress. Are you planning meals that require more time to prepare than you realistically have available? Is your family inadvertently hindering your efforts to follow the plan? Have you forgotten to purchase the necessary ingredients for specific meals?

Q. What if I struggle to find activities that match the feeling food gives me?
A. Don't worry if you initially can't seem to find activities that replicate the emotions you associate with food. It's entirely expected, given your deep-seated connection with food. The key is to select activities that hold personal significance for you. When engaging in these activities, make a conscious effort to fully immerse yourself in and appreciate the experience. Over time, as you continue substituting food

with meaningful activities, you'll notice a gradual shift. These activities will start to fulfil your emotional needs, simultaneously reducing food's grip on you and enhancing the perceived value of engaging in these new pursuits. This transformation will occur naturally as you continue with your efforts.

Q. What if I struggle to grasp emotional management without professional help?
A. This is a valid worry and was a primary consideration when writing this book. The chapters on mindset are designed to be structured and understandable, enabling individuals to grasp the concepts and the actions needed for success. Examples are provided to illustrate how to execute the exercises effectively. However, if you find that you still require additional guidance, there are resources available. Coaching services are an option, providing personalised support to assist you on your journey. Additionally, you can explore the online support group recommended on the *www.FoodFeelingsFreedom.com.au* website. There, you can connect with others facing similar challenges, gain insights, and receive assistance to manage your emotions.

<u>Something to think about:</u>

- Attempt to describe the food you consume. Use all of your five senses—sight, hearing, smell, taste, and touch.

- Contemplate how you would go about planning your meals for a fortnight. What would you need to consider?

- Think about and select activities that could serve as rewards or pick-me-ups.

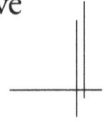

4

Food: Back to Basics

Throughout history, our connection with food has gone through remarkable transformations. Back in the days of the hunter/gatherers, food was a matter of survival. As civilisation advanced, the wealthy and noble would throw extravagant banquets that lasted for days, showcasing their prosperity and revelling in the celebration. And even today, many cultural traditions embrace the act of welcoming guests with food and drink.

But let's zoom in on the present. Food has evolved far beyond its role as a mere source of sustenance. It has become an integral part of our social interactions, carrying deep emotional significance. The exact reasons for this evolution are still a mystery, but some suggest that certain foods have been engineered to trigger the dopamine neurotransmitters in our brains, leaving us craving more. In regions with abundant food options and efficient transportation, convenience reigns supreme, making it easier than ever to satisfy our food desires.

With affluence on the rise and more time on our hands, we've found new ways to engage with food. While it has always been at the heart of celebrations and communal gatherings, recent decades have witnessed a gastronomic revolution. Talented cooks and chefs have turned food into a source of entertainment, captivating our senses through television shows and streaming platforms dedicated to culinary experiences.

Food holds a special place in our hearts, capable of conjuring up cherished memories and stirring powerful emotions. Think about tasting a dessert that takes you back to your childhood, where a single bite can transport you through time. These associations are widespread and widely accepted. However, for some individuals, food has become more than just nostalgia. It has become a coping mechanism—a go-to solution to manage emotions, regardless of their nature or intensity. This emotional bond with food, especially foods high in sugar, fat, and salt, triggers the area in the brain that is involved with pleasure and reward, releasing serotonin and dopamine chemicals when eaten. This *feel-good* feeling is a temporary relief and promotes calmness that, in turn, reduces the stress hormone cortisol. You may think this all sounds okay, but our minds and bodies do this over and over and become reliant on the comforting effects. As you give in to this dependency, your habits solidify, and the neural pathways in your brain strengthen, locking you into the cycle of emotional eating.

Escaping this cycle is no easy task. It requires a conscious decision and unwavering commitment to break free from deeply ingrained habits. While we won't delve into the complexities of neural pathways and the physical *withdrawal symptoms* that can occur, it's vital to recognise that reshaping your relationship with food is the key to liberating yourself from the grip of emotional eating. It's a journey of self-discovery and conscious choices, paving the way to a healthier and more balanced approach to nourishment.

A Perspective of Food

I'm all about finding clever shortcuts that make life smoother instead of wasting unnecessary effort. And let me tell you, when it comes to taking control of your relationship with food, this is one of those instances where working smarter truly pays off! The ultimate objective is to liberate yourself from the emotional grip food holds on you and establish a sustainable approach for the long haul.

In the previous chapter, we briefly explored the concept of shifting your perspective on food, unveiling two methods to reframe how you perceive it. You're absolutely on point in understanding that I'm asking you to consciously tweak your thoughts about food. It's a strategic manoeuvre that taps into the power of our minds, paving a clearer path toward achieving the desired outcome.

Now, as you embark on this transformation, it's vital to discover the strategies that mean something to you personally. We all have different approaches that click with us, and throughout the program, you'll actively embrace whatever works for you. Through consistent practice and dedication, by the program's end, you'll possess an understanding of which strategies deliver the most impactful results for you. It's all about finding what works for you and assembling a toolbox containing effective techniques that assist your journey towards having a healthier relationship with food.

Meal Planning

Meal planning is a game changer for so many reasons, with multiple benefits.

Firstly, let's consider logistics, like creating a plan, selecting ingredients, prepping food, and avoiding unnecessary waste. Whether you've used meal plans to save time or manage your weight, have you ever wondered why those plans are meticulously crafted? Some people have shared their thoughts, like how certain meal combinations offer specific health perks, nutrition experts advocate for dietary variety, and let's face it, following a ready-made plan is just plain easier. These insights are especially relevant to the goals of this program.

By following a meal plan, you can plan your meals ahead of time and stick to your food decisions. This lightens the load on your brain and reduces the mental effort required to figure out what to eat at every single meal. Many of us unknowingly spend heaps of mental energy each day contemplating, deciding, and planning our meals. To put it to the test, give this a trial. Have unplanned meals for three days, followed by three days of planned meals. Did you notice the difference in mental effort between the two approaches? Maybe you already know how much brain power you devote to thinking about food throughout the day.

Now, think about today. Are you thinking and planning your next meal even before you finish the one being eaten? When you follow a meal plan, you free up mental space. Instead of being constantly consumed by thoughts of food, you're liberated to focus on more fulfilling endeavours. You can choose what occupies your mind.

Let's discuss money - in particular, your food budget. Can you confidently set a specific amount of your budget for food and stick to it? Do you have a clear understanding of your actual food expenses? If you're an emotional eater, I suspect you may have a loose idea, but not really. And if you eat out a lot, you might not want to know how much you spend on food. If you're following or want to follow a budget, success can only come from creating and sticking to a plan that aligns with it.

Emotionally speaking, for those who grapple with emotional eating, meal planning comes to the rescue. By mapping out your meals in advance, you create a healthy emotional distance between your feelings and the food you consume. It's like downgrading the relationship from best friends to regular friends, as mentioned earlier when discussing the idea of friendships.

Considering the assortment of benefits, it's clear that meal planning is a practice that can work wonders for everyone, whether or not you're an emotional eater. It's a practical and empowering strategy that puts you in the driver's seat, allowing you to take control of your food choices and foster a healthier relationship with what you eat.

Food Rules

The specific food guidelines seamlessly complement meal planning. Rather than imposing strict rules on what you can or cannot eat, these guidelines revolve around narrowing down your range of food choices. This limitation aims to shift your perspective and intention regarding your upcoming meals. By consciously making deliberate decisions about your food choices, you heighten your awareness of what and why you're eating, steering clear of emotional eating tendencies. This intentional approach gradually weakens your emotional attachment to food.

One of the food rules is about limiting choice options. If I asked you to choose four different breakfasts that you can eat over the next two weeks, would you randomly pick four that immediately come to mind or would you think intentionally and consider factors like what your schedule is, whether you were going to be at home, or whether it can be a big or small breakfast, to list a few. You only have four options to eat from for the fortnight so make them nutritious, functional, realistic, and desirable. Remember, there isn't a restriction on the type of food; it's up to you what you eat. The restriction is the number of choices you give yourself.

Another crucial aspect of implementing these guidelines is creating a distinct environment around your food choices. The purpose is to foster a supportive atmosphere that aids in reshaping your current behaviours. It's about transforming how you engage with food and establishing a new normal that meets your desired outcomes. The main idea here is that if you want to adopt a new eating pattern, it's more effective if you follow a different routine, such as a meal plan with rules, rather than continuing to follow something that you're used to. Doing this reduces the chance of slipping back into old habits.

Exceptions

In both the program and in real life, unexpected surprises and uncontrollable situations are bound to happen. These moments call for you to focus on what works best for you in the here and now. If you cannot stick to the planned meals or follow the rules, don't worry. It's perfectly fine to acknowledge that you might need to hit the pause button on the program temporarily. You can always resume later or pick up where you left off once you regain control of your circumstances and can give the program the attention it requires.

Life is full of exceptions and curveballs. Anything can come your way, from work commitments and travel needs to family obligations, study deadlines, health concerns, financial worries, environmental issues, food shortages, and a whole array of challenging crises. It's vital to recognise that these circumstances can impact your ability to commit to the program fully. Remember, taking a breather or making necessary adjustments when the need arises is okay. What truly matters is that you prioritise your well-being and make choices that are realistic, appropriate, and consider the circumstances you're currently facing. Keep your focus on taking care of yourself and making the best decisions possible.

Eating Out

It's important to stay connected with friends, family, and colleagues during and after the program. If you get invited to hang out and have a good time, don't hesitate to say yes. In the past, food might have been the main event, stealing the spotlight from the awesome people you're with. But now, it's time for a shift. Instead of fixating on what's on your plate, let the focus be on the human company you're surrounded by. While you're following the program, your food choices when eating out are a bit more limited. Don't worry, though; it's all part of the plan. This way, you can still enjoy meals outside your home when necessary, but the real motivation is to enjoy the company of others.

To make this shift in mindset happen, we will shake things up a bit. Say goodbye to menu variety. The idea is to order the same thing every time you visit your favourite café or restaurant. Let's say you have a regular Wednesday lunch date at your local café and you have a few menu items you choose between. While on the program you will select menu items that will be your fixed choice for that venue. You can't change your mind, so pick something you're happy to eat repeatedly. If you like the Caesar salad then that will be the pick for that café. By keeping your menu selection consistent, the excitement and novelty of the food fades away, making it more like a background participant and a fuel rather than the main attraction. This way, you can truly enjoy the people you're with and the good times without the food stealing the show.

By following this rule, you can still socialise and enjoy yourself while also reaching the program's goal of breaking the emotional grip food can have on us. It's all about finding that sweet spot between enjoying social connections and maintaining a healthy relationship with food.

Food marketing cleverly taps into people's emotional attachment to food, skilfully moulding their purchasing decisions. They exploit this deep connection, manipulating individuals into indulging in their products while cleverly diverting attention from food being a basic nutritional energy source. How many "feeling" words do you see used in food marketing?

It feels incredibly unfair to be asked to strip away the emotions tied to our relationship with food and treat it like a cold, mechanical task. After all, food is more than just sustenance; it provides us with a profound sense of emotional comfort. So why would we willingly abandon something that brings us comfort, particularly when so many people rely on it for a mental health boost?

This, in itself, reveals a need for deep self-examination. It's clear that many individuals struggle to navigate their emotions effectively, a vital skill for nurturing our mental well-being. Consequently, they turn to food as a crutch, mistakenly believing it can fill the void and improve their mental state. Ironically, this reliance on food as a confidante only worsens the underlying issues, trapping them in a harmful, vicious cycle.

Nevertheless, if we can develop the ability to manage our emotions and make mindful choices about the foods we consume, we hold the key to breaking free from this destructive pattern. This newfound emotional intelligence grants us the power to embrace freedom and take control, enabling us to select the foods that truly bring us joy and nourishment.

These are some of the key elements involved in going back to basics with food:

- Changing your perspective of food
- Meal planning
- The rules about food

Changing Your Perspective of Food

Get ready to dive into the enlightening world of describing food. This activity demands your full attention, so pick a time when you can truly focus without distractions or time constraints. The goal here is to artfully describe the food you've chosen, leaving behind any judgments, emotional reactions, or societal opinions that may sway your perception.

Here's what you need to do:

1. Find a peaceful moment when you can immerse yourself in this activity without interruptions.

2. Take your pick of a single food item. Choose whatever you want, whether it's a piece of fruit, a biscuit, a chocolate bar, or a muesli bar.

3. Engage all five of your senses—sight, hearing, smell, taste, and touch—and vividly describe the chosen food item using your words.

4. Remember, this is all about describing, not evaluating. So resist the urge to judge the food item and focus solely on capturing its essence through your description.

Initially, you might find it a bit tricky to be perfectly literal in your descriptions. It takes practice and mindfulness to truly observe familiar foods without relying on assumptions. For instance, we rarely question the roundness of an orange because we instinctively recognise its ball-like shape. Describing the taste of an orange presents a challenge, as our brain tells us, "It tastes like an orange", or "It's orange flavoured". But how do we put that flavour into words? Expressing the sweetness, sourness, citrusy notes, or tanginess becomes an interesting struggle. Have you ever really paid attention to the textured skin of an orange? It's firm yet has cushiony dimples; it's slightly leathery or waxy to touch. Sometimes, we can't think of the vocabulary to capture these unique qualities, and maybe you'll have flashbacks to using adjectives in school English. Regardless, we all have different ideas and levels of language, so descriptions will vary from person to person. Be creative if you want, but the key here is to be descriptive.

Consider the word "healthy" when thinking about an orange. It doesn't describe any specific physical attributes related to appearance, sound, smell, taste, or touch. Rather, it's a label society uses to interpret and evaluate the qualities of an orange, implying that this food item is good for your health. Nutritionally, an orange is an orange; it is simply that.

As you diligently explore the food item with all your senses, you'll realise that it may take several minutes before you finally taste it. That's why it's crucial to allocate ample time for this process and avoid rushing through it. Once you've completed the activity, take a moment to reflect. Has your awareness and perspective of the food item transformed in any way? Were you able to resist the temptation to evaluate it? If you chose a *good* or *healthy* food item, assessing words might not have readily sprung to mind. However, assessing words might have surfaced if you chose to describe a chocolate bar or any item society deems unhealthy or fattening. For those who have ever been on a diet, their minds might be particularly adept at identifying *bad, unhealthy, fattening, treats*, or *naughty* foods, triggering evaluations whenever they attempt to choose or enjoy certain foods.

By immersing ourselves in a purely descriptive approach to food, we can eliminate all the evaluations and, in turn, lose the associated stigmas and emotions tied to each food item.

Meal Planning

The first step is to determine the specific meals to create a meal plan for the upcoming two weeks. The *Fortnight meal plan* worksheet, which can be copied from Chapter 12 or downloaded from the *www.FoodFeelingsFreedom.com.au* website, can help you in this process.

When creating your meal plan, keep the following important factors in mind:

- Consider whether the plan caters for your entire family or if it will be designed solely for yourself.
- Take a close look at your schedule for this period. Account for work, study, social engagements, and any travel plans.
- Assess your availability and energy levels when it comes to meal preparation. Identify the moments when you'll have the time and motivation to cook.
- Explore the option of pre-preparing some meals in advance, allowing for greater convenience during busy days.
- Take into consideration the capacity of your fridge and freezer, ensuring you have ample space to store your prepared meals.
- For those who are not in control of the household meal preparation, are you having separate meals for the duration of the program?

This is an example of a fortnight meal plan:

- *More flexibility is required for the evening meals; therefore, breakfast and lunch choices will have limited options.*
- *Four breakfast choices: yogurt and fruit, cocoa pops, oat porridge, or an almond croissant.*
- *Four lunch options: a ham and cheese sandwich, a protein shake, chicken breast and salad, or an omelette.*
- *As for snacks and supper, the four choices are a bowl of ice cream, a muesli bar, a hot chocolate, or a handful of almonds and cashews.*
- *When eating out:*
  - *Gianni's café – the order will always be an iced coffee and a blueberry friand.*
  - *Red Dragon Chinese restaurant – the order will be Mongolian beef, seasonal vegetables with oyster sauce, jasmine rice, and a glass of Sauvignon Blanc.*
  - *Spicy Indian – the order will be butter chicken and peshwari naan.*

Take the above factors into account as you decide on your flexible meals. To ensure a successful plan, prioritise simplicity, opt for dishes you want to eat, minimise effort, and maintain a realistic approach. Remember, your choices don't necessarily have to revolve around healthiness; you can address that aspect later if it aligns with your goals. Make a firm decision to commit to your plan, and no excuses!

Here are some insightful tips shared by individuals who have completed this program:

- *Dedicate time on weekends to prepare meals in advance.*
- *Ensure you have a wide range of meals in sufficient quantities to last for the entire two weeks.*
- *Consider the size of your freezer when determining the amount and variety of prepared meals you want to store.*
- *Plan meals that can easily be reheated on days when time or energy for cooking is limited.*
- *Include a meal option that your family can reheat or manage on days when you're working late.*
- *Explore the convenience of purchasing restaurant food and freezing it in portion-sized servings.*
- *Save the free main meal for a Saturday, aligning it with your socialising or relaxation time.*

Take a moment to reflect on these suggestions and observe what would work best for you as you progress through your planning and implementation over the coming weeks. Remember, the key is to commit to your plan without making changes. However, it's helpful to make notes or keep a record of how you manage your food choices throughout the week, allowing for adjustments in future fortnight plans.

Food Rules

These are the rules for the fortnight meal plan:

1. You cannot change your mind once you decide on your choices.
2. Decide when your flexible meal will be. Is it the morning, midday or the evening meal?
3. The flexible meal can include a different choice every day, or you can repeat some meals if you want; the choice is yours.
4. For the other meals of the day, you are restricted to a maximum of four options for each of them.
5. If you have morning tea, afternoon tea or supper, these are collectively called 'snacks', and you can choose a maximum of four options in total.
6. Order the same menu per premises if you're eating out.
7. From week 5, allocate *unplanned flexible meals* per week.

Frequently Asked Questions:

Q: I'm feeling a bit lost when it comes to changing my mindset about food. Where should I start?
A: To shift your focus towards food, it's essential to build awareness of what you eat. If you find it overwhelming at first, a great entry point is meal planning—it's a more

approachable step. By actively participating in meal planning and making conscious decisions about your food choices, you'll gradually develop a heightened sense of awareness. As this awareness grows, you'll have the power to alter your perspective on each food item you encounter.

Q: My work schedule is unpredictable, and I can't commit to planning meals for a full fortnight. What should I do?
A: If you find the idea of planning meals for two weeks too daunting, don't worry. You can still create a plan that works for you by focusing on a week instead. The same principles apply but with a bit more flexibility. Remember, even a modified plan is better than no plan at all.

If a week still feels like a stretch and you're determined to regain control over emotional eating, consider planning for four days instead. Give yourself two choices for restricted meals during this period. And here's the secret: you can repeat the same week or four-day plan multiple times to achieve the desired outcome. The key here is adaptability. Find a strategy that suits your unpredictable schedule and helps you to take charge of your meals.

Q: Why are the food rules so important?
A: The food rules play a crucial role in our journey towards a healthier relationship with food. They serve two significant purposes. Firstly, they encourage food awareness by prompting us to think consciously and make deliberate decisions about our food choices for the fortnight. Through

this process, we become more attuned to what we eat and how it impacts our well-being. Secondly, the food rules serve as a powerful tool for behavioural change. Breaking away from our old patterns and embracing new guidelines disrupts the status quo and creates space for positive transformations. The rules act as a catalyst, shifting our mindset and helping us focus on making sustainable and beneficial changes in our eating habits.

Something to think about:

- If you were to create a meal plan, would you choose breakfast, lunch or the evening meal to be the flexible meal?

- How can you make the fortnight plan simple so that you can succeed?

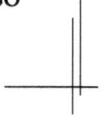

5

Activities: It's Time To Do

This program component is a substitute crutch, replacing your dependence on food with a different kind of support. It is still a behavioural alternative, something you can physically do because, let's face it, it's easier to take action than to reshape thoughts. If you face a daunting task and are fighting procrastination, instead of diving into the challenge headfirst and pushing through the discomfort, you find yourself raiding the pantry for a snack. It's more appealing to choose an activity that brings joy, like playing with a dog or listening to music, than to put yourself through mental suffering.

Engaging in activities is the most obvious substitute for a crutch, as it offers natural alternatives with numerous benefits. The possibilities are endless, limited only by our imagination, accessibility, and finances. While some activities may have negative consequences, you have the power to choose positive and fulfilling options. It doesn't matter what your circumstances are, you can create a personalised list of unique activities.

Speaking of variety, the options are practically infinite. You can get creative and design your own activities. Think about what holds the most significant meaning for you, considering your unique circumstances and available resources. Do you need some inspiration? Then check out a comprehensive list in Chapter 12. Do any of these activities interest you? Immersing yourself in a chapter of a book, taking a 20-minute stroll outdoors or along the beach, sharing 15 minutes with an animal companion, doing a 30-minute craft project, indulging in an episode of TV or streaming series, treating yourself to a movie, spending 30 minutes scrolling through social media, dedicating 30 minutes to any hobby that brings you joy, or engaging in a 15-minute conversation with a friend or neighbour. The possibilities are as vast as your imagination and the resources at your disposal.

The activity list isn't some rigid daily checklist you must complete. It stands apart from the daily task lists some people create. If you're a fan of daily must-do lists, maintain that, but I also encourage you to develop an activity list. The activity list comes into play when you find yourself experiencing the emotions you used to manage by turning to food. Once you recognise those familiar feelings, turn to your activity list instead, exploring alternative actions to replace the old habit. You may not tick off every activity in a single day, but that's alright. The list is a living, breathing entity that evolves over time. Add new options and cross off completed activities—think of it as a dynamic companion that adapts to your changing needs.

With progress and time, you'll reach a point where you can manage your emotions without relying on activities as a crutch. You may even discover that you genuinely enjoy many chosen activities for their inherent benefits and the positive emotions they evoke.

Activity Rules

The rules for each activity are designed with two crucial factors in mind: duration and frequency. These guidelines exist to ensure that we maintain our interest, enjoyment, and enthusiasm for the activity. It may seem counterintuitive, as one would assume that engaging in an enjoyable activity every day would sustain our excitement for it. However, our brain chemistry tells a different story. Initially, when we venture into something new, we experience the greatest pleasure. Yet, as we repeatedly engage in the activity over time, our interest gradually diminishes.

Have you ever stumbled upon a new hobby or interest and completely immersed yourself in it, only to find the initial spark fading away? Perhaps you indulged in a marathon of a TV series, finishing it within a week, and felt a sense of emptiness afterwards, wondering what to watch next. It might have taken some time to regain that level of interest or find another captivating show. Do you remember when a television show was shown weekly and you waited impatiently for that day to arrive? Your anticipation was maintained for weeks, months and even years! The same pattern applies to social media. If we mindlessly scroll for hours each day, our overall interest wanes, and we constantly seek fresh content to keep us engaged. Notably, social media companies are well aware of this brain response and actively provide new material to counteract the saturation of our interest.

By imposing limitations on our experiences with activities, we can preserve our enthusiasm and extend our enjoyment of them.

Exceptions

In both the program and life, unexpected circumstances and events beyond our control are bound to happen. During these times, it becomes crucial to prioritise what is most suitable for you at that particular moment. If you cannot follow the activity rules, it's essential to acknowledge this reality and explore alternative options. Consider temporarily pausing the program, seeking guidance from a counsellor to explore alternative approaches, then resuming when you can regain control over the situation or prioritise the program requirements. It's important to understand that certain exceptions may arise due to various factors such as work commitments, travel or family obligations, time constraints, health or financial concerns, environmental factors, or any other challenging crises that may impact your ability to commit to the program fully.

I understand that you might find it frustrating that I'm suggesting replacing one crutch with another instead of immediately addressing the root issue of managing your emotions. However, it's essential to recognise that learning to navigate and control our emotions is a gradual process that requires time and practice. Just like mastering the art of walking before attempting to run, taking a slow and steady approach while following the program can significantly enhance your chance of success.

If you strongly feel inclined to bypass the activities component, you can do so, but it's crucial to ensure you have a robust support system in place. This may involve seeking guidance from a mental health professional, connecting with a supportive community or support group, or relying on individuals who can offer specific assistance to help you transition towards managing your emotions without relying on a crutch.

This chapter will look at the three main aspects of creating an activities list:

1. Selecting activities for specific purposes
2. General activities
3. Expanding your interests

Selecting Activities for Specific Purposes

If you need help deciding where to dive in, Chapter 12 has got you covered with a comprehensive list of activity ideas. Take your time looking through the list and discover the ones that spark some interest in you.

Whether you're seeking a well-deserved reward, a comforting escape, stress relief, a remedy for procrastination, or simply a cure for boredom, the options are endless. No longer will food be your sole companion in these moments. Instead, you're introducing various activities to keep your enthusiasm and curiosity alive.

If you have specific reasons, handpick at least four activities that truly resonate with you, which hold personal meaning and will bring you joy. These chosen activities will help you navigate these emotional situations. And remember, if you find yourself encountering these reasons frequently, don't hesitate to expand your list to six or more activities per reason.

Selecting General Activities

When dealing with emotions outside of the specific ones mentioned above, you have a wide range of activities from the general list to choose from. These activities don't necessarily have to be as enjoyable or personally meaningful as the specific ones. They can be any activity that you're open to trying.

Select a minimum of six activities for the general list. Feel free to be curious and experiment with different options. And remember, you have the freedom to expand your collection of activities as you see fit. The ultimate aim is to have a diverse list of activities that are available to help you navigate and help manage a variety of emotional states.

Allow me to introduce you to Michael and provide a glimpse into his initial selection of activities.

Michael is fifty years old, married with three grown children, and very involved with his grandchildren. He works full-time in a government office and in his personal time, indulges in his hobbies of camping, fishing, cooking, and entertaining family and friends.

Now, let's take a look at Michael's personalised activity list, which showcases his unique choices and offers an example:

Activity List

Plan next camping trip

Find new camping recipes

Learn the guitar

Listen to music

Organise the shed

Learn to read music

Look at social media

Landscaping the backyard

   - BBQ area

   - Gazebo

   - Vegetable garden

   - Pond area

   - Irrigation

To reward myself

Look at fishing content on You Tube

Watch 4WD show on television

Play with the grandchildren

Go fishing

When I am ... Frustrated

Go for a walk

Mow the grass

Weed the garden

Wash the car

To comfort myself

Listen to old Rock music

Sit with the dogs

Talk to a friend

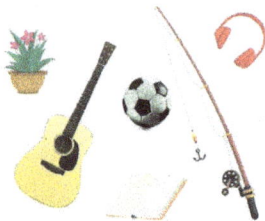

Other ... when feeling down

Look at photos from past camping trips

Talk to my wife

Expanding Your Interests

When creating your personal list of activities, it's only natural to lean towards the familiar and comfortable options - activities you're already acquainted with and enjoy. But I want to challenge you to break free from the confines of your usual choices. It's time to push the boundaries and explore new territories. Permit yourself to select activities that ignite your curiosity, and consider activities that have lingered on your wish list for far too long. You can take on a larger project and break it down into bite-sized, manageable tasks that you can complete over weeks or months.

Let's draw inspiration from Michael's journey. Michael had always nurtured a secret desire to learn a musical instrument. So, he embraced the challenge and added learning the guitar to his general list of activities. Furthermore, he dreamed about transforming his garden into a beautiful oasis. Instead of overwhelming himself with the entire project, Michael wisely chose to list the smaller components of the landscaping on his general list. He understood there was no need to rush; he could tackle each element at his own pace, following the prescribed rules.

The Rules

1. Each activity can be done once or a maximum of twice per week.

2. Activities are time-limited.
   - Do any activity/hobby for up to 30 minutes
   - If the activity has a natural endpoint, then stop at that time
   - Watch one episode of a TV/streaming show, a maximum of 1 hour
   - Watch a movie until it finishes
   - If you're reading a book, finish the chapter close to the 30-minute time limit
3. From week 7, the Activity rules are relaxed (this is optional).

Frequently Asked Questions:

Q. What if I'm too busy to engage in non-essential activities?
A. Once you liberate yourself from the constant preoccupation with food, you'll unlock time to explore other fulfilling endeavours that you didn't have time for before. There will be occasions when you want comfort or crave a reward, presenting the opportunity to replace your reliance on food with alternative activities. Instead of grabbing a handful of biscuits, look at your list and see what you could do.

Q. I'm not keen on choosing activities to participate in. Can I skip this part?
A. I hear you, and it's understandable to feel hesitant about this aspect of the program. However, it's important to recognise the significance of replacing the food crutch

with another behavioural alternative as you work towards mastering emotional self-management. While skipping this component is an option, if you do, I highly recommend you seek counselling support for the initial eight weeks of the program. This guidance can help and support you so you can transition towards managing your emotions without relying on a crutch.

Q. Why don't I feel the same excitement or satisfaction from activities as I did from using food for reward or comfort?
A. It's natural to wonder about the difference in emotional impact between activities and food. Food has been a trusted companion, offering comfort and joy in various situations. Think of it like friendship: food is your best friend, providing intense emotions when celebrating or seeking comfort. On the other hand, activities are more like regular friends, offering enjoyment but not quite reaching the same level of intensity.

However, as you gradually reduce the importance of food in your life, the value and anticipated benefits of activities will begin to balance out. It's a process of changing your emotional associations and developing new patterns. Over time, you'll discover that engaging in activities can bring a sense of fulfilment and satisfaction. You'll find alternative ways to reward yourself and seek comfort beyond food.

Something to think about:

- What activities would you put on your *Activity list*?

- What activities would you choose to reward or comfort you?

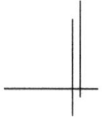

6

The Power of the Mind

When you experience emotions, there's often a chance that your feelings will be visible. For instance, when you feel nervous, people will notice your fidgeting, trembling hands, flushed face, shaky voice, or even visibly sweating. Similarly, if anger grips you, your face might turn red, have a stormy expression, and your arms and hands may tense up and be clenched.

When it comes to thoughts and the ability to know what's on someone's mind, it can get tricky. Some thoughts may leak out through facial expressions, tones of voice, posture, or physical appearance, especially if someone is expressive. But it's often easier to hide our thoughts from others. How often have you spoken or acted in a way, while thinking something entirely different, and nobody knew what you were thinking? This becomes a problem when you attempt to change a habit or embark on something new. You may start with the best intentions and motivations, but if your mind decides to be stubborn, it could come up with excuses, delay your efforts, or conjure up any number of reasons to frustrate your progress. This internal battle with your thoughts often goes unnoticed by others. Some people might share a similar experience, but nobody truly knows the intricate workings of your mind.

This is precisely why it's often easier to engage in activities, make plans, or modify your behaviour than to change how you think. Since thoughts are invisible, we can't observe whether change occurs or measure success. This lack of control of our thoughts is why some people hesitate when faced with programs that aim to alter thought patterns. Fighting against your mind can be an uphill battle, and no one can truly fathom the mental obstacle course your mind can present. Without external accountability, our minds can craft sneaky ways to undermine our efforts, potentially leading to another failed attempt.

Avoiding Discomfort

Have you ever noticed how you try to avoid certain emotions while actively seeking out others? For instance, if being the centre of attention makes you uncomfortable, you'll go to great lengths to dodge speaking in front of a group. When faced with an impending deadline, you might procrastinate on your task until the absolute last moment. And if you're someone who shies away from confrontations, the idea of having difficult conversations fills you with dread, and you'll do anything to avoid them.

Even without consciously realising it, we often strive to minimise or sidestep uncomfortable thoughts and feelings. We willingly resort to distractions, denial, postponement, or self-negotiation to steer ourselves toward feeling more comfortable. For instance, you might opt for email communication if you'd prefer not to engage with someone in person. You might even choose to forgo a job promotion to avoid the nervousness that comes with a job interview. Boring or uncomfortable tasks? You'll allow yourself to be side-tracked until the last minute.

The specific thoughts and emotions that make us uncomfortable vary from person to person. You can usually identify them by the circumstances or situations you go out of your way to avoid or by your reliance on coping mechanisms, such as food.

We tend to label the things we dislike as *bad* or *negative*. This same tendency applies to uncomfortable thoughts and emotions; we often perceive them as undesirable and something we should eliminate or evade. Conversely, we label enjoyable and welcomed thoughts and feelings as *good* and *positive*. Recall our previous discussion about food, where we learned to literally describe it and treat food as fuel rather than categorising it as *good, bad, naughty,* or *healthy.* Similarly, feelings and emotions are essentially thoughts created by your mind and emotions can be felt in your mind and body. They can also be described in neutral terms, and terms like *good, bad, positive,* or *negative* are subjective evaluations that shape our reactions.

If you notice yourself feeling nervous, take a moment to reflect on the thoughts running through your mind and how your body responds. When stepping into something new or striving to make a positive impression, it's normal to experience nervousness because you genuinely care about the situation. Feeling uncomfortable is a natural part of this process and doesn't inherently signify something bad or negative. You don't have to relish uncomfortable thoughts or feelings; it's perfectly fine not to enjoy them. However, if you're controlling your situations to avoid discomfort, it's worth considering that your actions are working against your overall well-being. If this rings true, and you desire a change, seeking support from a mental health professional can be a valuable step to help you navigate these challenges.

From a practical perspective, it can look like this:
Casper admitted they didn't like clothes shopping. They didn't like the process of trying on clothes to ensure they fit, engaging with shop attendants and admitting that fashionable clothes on the racks didn't fit. As a result of feeling uncomfortable and discouraged, they would buy clothes online, often buying clothes that didn't fit and wasting money. Instead of facing up to how

they felt and doing something to change the situation, they went with the flow, and their behaviour continued.

Let's reach for the sky here… what do you avoid doing because you don't want unpleasant or uncomfortable feelings and emotions?

When you experience typical emotions that often trigger emotional eating, such as anxiety, sadness, frustration, boredom, hopelessness, or stress, these emotions prompt specific thoughts and sensations in your mind and body. By consciously describing these thoughts and feelings and not evaluating them, you can retrain your brain to interpret and respond to them differently, ultimately leading to changes in your behaviour.

The Cheer Squad

You've probably come across stories of people achieving remarkable things in the face of adversity. Perhaps you even have a personal connection to someone who embodies that determined spirit. So, how does this happen, and how can you make it happen for you? This is a question that often arises, especially when you find yourself falling victim to self-sabotage, derailing your own intentions time and time again.

Believe it or not, achieving something extraordinary is within your grasp if you approach it with positive belief, persistence, motivation and a firm grounding in reality. The path to success may be riddled with daunting hills and unexpected curves, but when you genuinely believe in your ability to reach your goal, your mind seizes onto something tangible. It's like having your very own cheer squad built right into your thoughts that fuels your determination. Believing in yourself doesn't guarantee a smooth and obstacle-free ride. It simply means that with your unwavering conviction, you can persist and overcome any hurdles that dare to come your way.

This realistic and unwavering belief is a deeply personal and unique experience that resides within you. Your mind forms the bond with your dreams, so if others deem your goals unrealistic or unattainable, that's their business. Let their scepticism be their burden while you remain steadfast in pursuing your dreams. This is your journey, and you can shape it based on your own solid belief.

When we're on our own, we often devise countless excuses to dodge discomfort. The support of people around you is crucial to staying on course and holding yourself accountable for your goals. You can achieve things on your own, relying on your own belief, but it is easier if you have people encouraging you along the way.

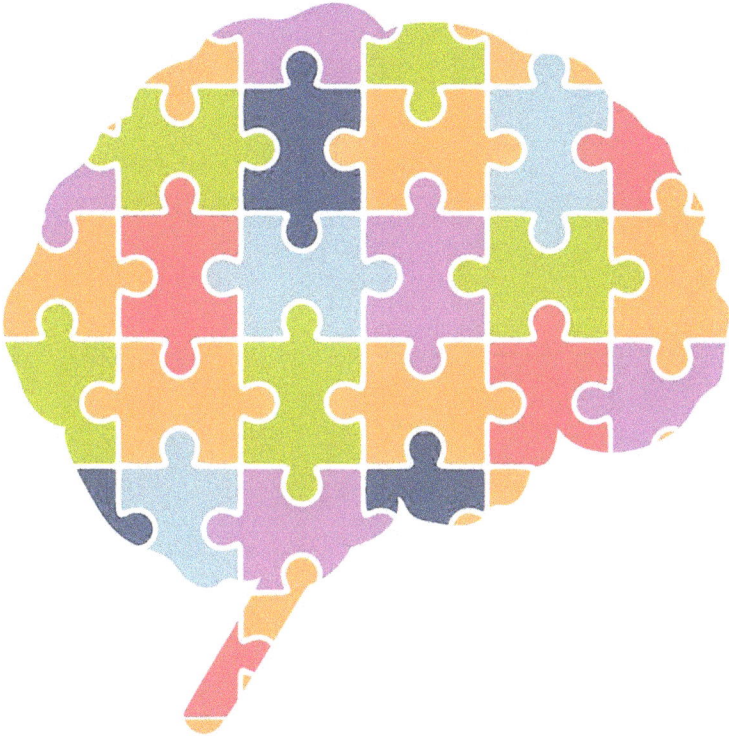

These are the steps involved in examining the key pieces to understanding and managing your emotional mind:

- Emotional awareness
- Acknowledge and identify bodily sensations
- Describe emotions
- Choose to experience emotions
- Take control

Emotional Awareness

Awareness and understanding of your feelings and emotions form the foundation of a fascinating journey. We're not just talking about the obvious big feelings like anger, sadness, and happiness; we're diving deep into the realm of more subtle emotions, too.

Let's practice recognising your emotions as they arise. Here's what to do:

- Tune in to what you're feeling.
- Identify what sparked it.
- Take note of the thoughts racing through your mind.
- Recognise how you reacted in that moment.

You can focus on any of these aspects and in any order to get started. The key is bringing a thought, feeling, sensation, or reaction into your mind. It might not immediately make sense why you're thinking, feeling, or reacting a certain way, but simply acknowledging something is happening is the first step. You can choose to think about these observations, or you can write them down. Do whatever works best for you.

For those struggling with emotional eating, this practice can be particularly insightful. If you reach for food without knowing why, chances are some underlying emotion drives that behaviour. Except, of course, when you're genuinely

hungry – that's perfectly normal. You can use the *Food &
Feelings Diary* worksheet provided to identify the emotions
linked to your eating habits. It's essential to break the
automatic association between emotions and food. We
often turn to the pantry out of boredom, nervousness, or
procrastination without realising that these actions are rooted
in emotions. By becoming more aware of these connections,
you can disentangle your feelings from your eating habits.

Remember, emotional awareness is a gradual process, and
it's okay if you don't catch everything at once. The key is to
stay curious and attentive to your feelings, and with time
and practice, you'll develop a deeper understanding of your
emotional landscape.

Acknowledge and Identify Bodily Sensations

When you feel emotions bubbling up inside you, take a
moment and pay attention to what you're feeling. What
captures your attention first? Is it the emotional sensation,
bodily reactions, or automatic reactions and behaviour? You
can either grab a notebook or print out the *Think Feel Body
Connection* worksheet to start unravelling the inner workings
of your mind and body when emotions arise.

Think of this as a "feeling" puzzle. You'll gradually assemble
the pieces, and the whole picture will eventually emerge.
Some of these pieces may take time to surface, but that's

precisely why we go through the various steps in this program.

Some might feel bodily sensations, such as a tight, overwhelming pressure in their chest or an uncomfortable knot in their stomach, but that's as far as it goes. They may not be aware of their thoughts or behaviour at that moment, and connecting it all to the emotion they're experiencing can be challenging. This is where some people begin when piecing together the puzzle. It requires time and a willingness to pay attention and be open to your feelings and thoughts.

Others may recognise a specific feeling, such as nervousness, but they might not see the link with the other components. We all have unique ways of understanding and learning about our emotions. Hence, there's no fixed starting point. What matters is the desire to acknowledge and identify all the pieces.

If you believe you're already in touch with the feelings and emotions you experience, write each on a *Think Feel Body Connection* worksheet. Ensure you don't overlook any pieces; they are all important in revealing how that feeling unfolds in your mind, body, and behaviour. While the worksheet doesn't have a dedicated space for documenting your behaviours or reactions, feel free to write them anywhere on the page.

Think, Feel, Body Connection

When I'm feeling

Irritated

(Annoyed, frustrated)

These are some of my thoughts

- I want to do things that I want to do.
- I am tired.
- These people annoy me.
- This is wasting my time.
- Why has this gone wrong
- Get me out of here.

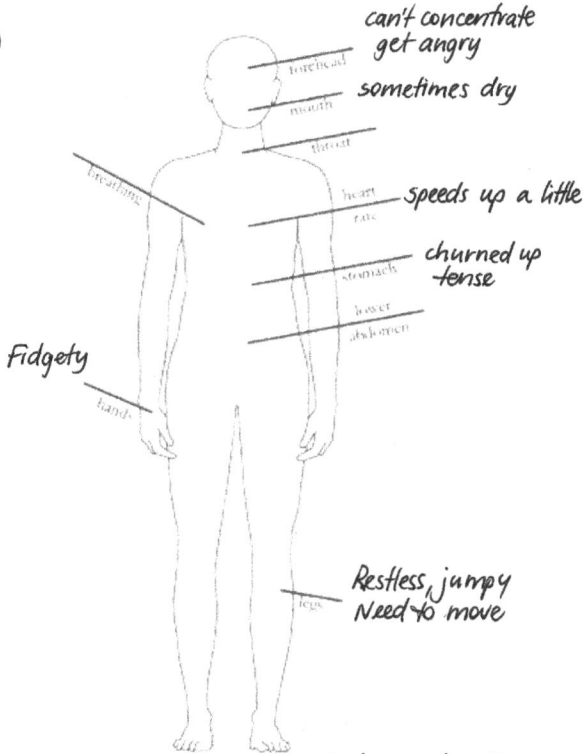

can't concentrate
get angry
forehead
sometimes dry
mouth

throat

breathing

heart rate — speeds up a little

stomach — churned up
tense

lower abdomen

Fidgety

hands

Restless, jumpy
Need to move
legs

Behaviour - sometimes need to leave situations
- sometimes rude to people

* The idea is that you identify the emotion you feel, what thoughts you're having and where you feel body sensations
- cut people off from talking

Describe Emotions

Now that you've started tuning in to your feelings and noticing the physical sensations in your body, the next step involves describing what's happening. Just as you've learned

103

to describe food in neutral terms rather than assigning value labels, now you'll do the same for how your emotions affect your mind and body.

Here's an example from Lexa when she felt tired:

- *Mind: was fuzzy like cotton wool and difficult to think*
- *Arms and legs: felt heavy as if they were each carrying a weight*
- *Eyes and eyelids: droopy and challenging to keep eyes open*

We often tend to categorise anything uncomfortable as negative or bad and something to avoid. After all, how could something causing discomfort possibly be good? This thinking stems from associating value judgments with actions and feelings, therefore shaping our perception. To simplify, an emotion is just an emotion; it can come with associated thoughts, feelings, and sensations. Our fear of discomfort, family upbringing, or societal norms has influenced whether we think it's good or bad.

During this exercise of describing what's happening in your mind and body, the challenge lies in not automatically labelling the emotion as good or bad. View the feeling for what it literally is without the added value label. If you're still finding it difficult to describe emotions without evaluating them, don't worry; you can pause here and spend some extra time on this step, or you can continue and see if the following exercise helps clear things up for you. If you've got the hang of it, then full steam ahead.

Choose to Experience Emotions

What if I asked you to welcome your emotions with open arms, explore them, and be curious about their impact? Are you a bit unsure? Regardless of the displayed emotion: fear, nervousness, anger, excitement, stress, or any other feeling, take a moment to observe the thoughts they trigger, the bodily sensations they create, and how you instinctively want to respond. Think of it like stepping into a lolly store, where you want to sample all the different flavours. Some you might find pleasant, others not so much, but it's about the experience of trying them all.

When you're experiencing the emotion, be curious about the associated bodily sensations, your thoughts and instinctive behaviour. You're not judging or evaluating the emotion, just being curious. If your emotions are intense and you find it hard to stay curious and know what is going on inside you, don't stress. Start by practising during times when your emotions are weaker. As you practise and get better at dealing with your feelings, you'll find it easier to experience and handle stronger emotions.

Intense emotions might hit you, particularly if you feel overwhelmed and engulfed in the emotion, or when you're aware that a known stressful situation will trigger you. As you get better at handling your emotions, you will be able to navigate intense thoughts and emotions and still be able to function, both physically and mentally. If you need assistance with intense emotions, seek help from a mental health professional.

Take Control

As you approach the destination of your journey to understand and manage emotions, let's consolidate everything you've learned. You're now more than 80% of the way there. When an emotion strikes, it's important to process it objectively and explore its impact on your thoughts, feelings, and bodily sensations. Regardless of the emotion and intensity, it is possible to think clearly and function as needed. With this heightened emotional awareness, you can introduce a powerful concept called reframing. It involves identifying your thoughts, feelings, or reactions and seeing them from a different perspective.

Allow me to illustrate this with an example:

> *Michael frequently felt frustrated, bored, and unhappy during workdays. On such occasions, he'd turn to snacks and his favourite lunches to give himself something to look forward to. As he became more attuned to his underlying emotions, he began swapping his food fixes*

with other activities that could be done at work. By diving deeper into his feelings, he learned to identify them and understand how they influenced his thoughts, feelings, and behaviours. At this point, he focused on the thoughts that led to his frustration and boredom. Most of these thoughts revolved around not understanding why he was assigned specific tasks and why colleagues with less experience received preferential treatment.

Michael had two options if he wanted to improve his emotional state:

1. **Change his thought patterns:** He could reframe his thoughts to create a more positive outlook. Instead of saying, "This task is not challenging for me," he could say, "I have sufficient knowledge and skills for this task".

2. **Take action:** Michael could address the situation with his manager.

Michael spoke to his manager about being considered for higher responsibilities or a promotion. In the meantime, he altered his thought patterns, which enabled him to find satisfaction in his work. This shift in thinking had a ripple effect on his overall mood and improved his interactions with colleagues. Reflecting on his previous reliance on snacks and lunches to cope, Michael discovered he no longer needed or desired them to get through the day.

It's essential to recognise that even when circumstances are beyond your control, you still have power over your thoughts. While trying to find a positive spin on something that contradicts reality might seem counterintuitive, you can always believe in yourself. Repeatedly telling yourself positive affirmations like "I am strong," "I am resilient," or "I have the knowledge I need" can make a significant impact on your emotional well-being.

Frequently Asked Questions:

Q. What do I do when I am overwhelmed or caught by an emotion?
A. Take proactive steps if you recognise situations or triggers that overwhelm you emotionally. First, identify these triggers or situations. Then, work on developing a plan to prevent yourself from becoming overwhelmed. Practise this plan and implement it as soon as you notice the initial signs of being triggered. You may need assistance from a mental health professional if this is too difficult for you to do by yourself.

Q. I understand the steps but struggle to understand what's happening within me.
A. It's perfectly normal not to see what's happening with ourselves sometimes. Others who observe our behaviour often see things we can't. If you find yourself in this situation, consider seeking support from a trusted friend, a

peer in an online support group, a coach, or a mental health professional.

Q. Must I follow all the steps in this chapter?
A. You're not obligated to go through all of them if you're already familiar and skilled in these stages. In such cases, feel free to skip to the step you need. However, suppose you're uncertain about your emotions and their impact on your mind and body. In that case, the step-by-step approach outlined here will lead you towards understanding those emotions, what to do about them, and improve your emotional management.

Something to think about

- Can you name the emotions you feel?

- Do you feel bodily sensations when you're emotional?

- What emotions do you find uncomfortable? Do you take steps to avoid situations that provoke them?

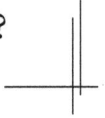

7

Monitoring Your Progress: Is It Working?

Whenever we engage in any activity, we always want to know how we are progressing and whether we're on the right track. This in itself helps us stay motivated so we can continue with whatever we're doing. The same applies to following the suggestions in this book and program. How do you know that what you're doing is right and whether it is helping you progress to what you want to achieve?

Setting Goals

Let's talk about what you want to achieve and turn those aspirations into tangible goals. Setting goals can be a bit tricky because sometimes you're not exactly sure what you want; instead, you might know what you don't want. Other times, the goal you have in mind is so broad and undefined that it's hard to know when you've actually reached it. Think back to why you picked up this book in the first place. Did it spark thoughts about your life and things you want to change? This is the starting point for understanding where you are now and where you want to go.

To get there, take some time to explore your thoughts and behaviours. Evaluate how they impact your life and decide if there's anything you want to change. Visit the *www. FoodFeelingsFreedom.com.au* website for a downloadable *Goal-setting* worksheet, or feel free to record your goals in a way that suits you. Whether you use the worksheet or a notepad to create your goals, make sure to follow the SMART goal approach, ensuring they are specific enough for you to recognise when you've achieved them. Once you've created your goals, write them on the *Goal-o-meter* worksheet. Use this when you check in on your progress; it lets you visualise your progress on the scale.

If reflecting on yourself is new to you, it might take a bit of time to grasp what I'm asking. Perhaps you've realised you have an issue with food, and it's causing problems, but pinpointing what comes next is challenging. Don't worry; you can talk to a program buddy, join a support group, or consult a health professional to help clarify your goals. Alternatively, you can identify specific issues and work on reducing or minimising them.

Let's break down the main components of this process and get a general idea of each one.

Your perception of food

You're no longer caught up in constant thoughts about food or constantly planning meals. You become more at ease with what food represents, seeing it simply as a source of nourishment you choose to enjoy. It stops being the central focus when you socialise; instead, it takes a back seat, allowing you to connect with people more meaningfully.

Breaking it down:
- You've developed a meal plan that's easy to follow.
- You've learnt what works for you and your circumstances.
- Planning meals within certain guidelines doesn't feel limiting anymore.
- You've accepted that food is not the main attraction during social activities.
- Your perspective on food has evolved—it's now seen as a vital fuel source for your body. You don't rely on it to cope with your emotions. You have a higher regard for food because you appreciate what it gives your body.
- Describing food based on its literal qualities takes the emotional baggage away from food. You don't feel guilty about eating or drinking something of your choice.

Discovering your interests and hobbies

Make the most of your time and mental energy by engaging in activities you truly enjoy, even those you couldn't do before. Embracing a variety of activities enriches your life, opening up new possibilities. As you invest time in these activities, you'll find that they become genuinely enjoyable and can extend beyond the program's completion. Regardless of how deeply rooted some of your emotional eating habits may be, you're gradually and successfully shifting your focus from food to these fulfilling activities.

Breaking it down:

- Be open to creating a large list of possible activities pending your resources and requirements.
- The rules don't feel limiting and support your desire to spread out your interests and activities; no more bingeing.
- Life is richer from all the additional interests you have pursued.

Your emotions

The first big step for anything related to your mental health and well-being is to be aware of, acknowledge, and manage your emotions. Knowing how you're progressing regarding your emotions is very individualistic. Everyone could have a different starting position and may progress in their own unique way. If you're doing this program with a buddy, remember that you'll each be on your own path, even though there will be shared experiences along the way.

Breaking it down:
- Become aware of feeling emotions.
- Including all the emotion puzzle pieces – recognising them, giving them a name, what thoughts are associated with them, how they present themselves within your body e.g. bodily sensations, how you react with them, and what causes them in the first place.
- You are able to describe and not judge the emotion being felt.
- Learning to welcome and wanting to experience emotions as opposed to running away or avoiding uncomfortable emotions.
- Knowing that some words, thoughts, people, or situations trigger emotions and working through how they can be managed in order to live life how you want.

Trial the Program

The structured progression of this program unfolds over 8 weeks. You can hit pause and stay at any point for as long as you need. This is particularly relevant after week 4, when we delve into the mindset component. If you feel comfortable and reach a desired level, you can stop following the individual components or take a break from the entire program.

An important part of having a break from the components or the program is to monitor your progress. Are you staying on course and working towards or maintaining your new goals, or are you slipping back into past habits? Monitoring means consciously comparing your current thoughts and behaviours with your desired goals.

Feel free to perform a thoughts or behaviour check whenever needed. For instance, if you identified that you turned to chocolate biscuits whenever you felt sad and needed a pick-me-up. If you notice that tendency re-occurring, it could signal that you might be slipping back into unwanted behaviours.

This is how you can monitor your progress throughout the program:

- Creating goals
- Key questions to ask yourself
- *FoodFeelingsFreedom* (3*F) quiz

Creating Goals

Perhaps you're familiar with the SMART concept for goal-setting, but if not, let's break it down. The five letters represent different aspects of this approach:

(S)	Specific	All the "W's" - who, what, when and why
(M)	Measurable	Determine how you'll know if you've reached your goal
(A)	Attainable	Ensure it's achievable
(R)	Relevant	Be honest about what you can realistically accomplish
(T)	Timely	Set a date or timeframe to keep yourself accountable

Consider these questions as you create your goals using the SMART approach:

Goal Setting

SPECIFIC • What do you want to achieve and WHY*?	*Reduce time thinking about food. I spend too much time thinking about food and planning meals which stops me from doing other things.*

*The WHY is important as it reinforces the reason behind your goal

MEASURABLE • How are you measuring the success of the goal	*Limit thoughts and planning to 10 minutes per snack or meal.*
ATTAINABLE • How important is this to you • Is this goal realistic	*It can be achieved by planning and sticking to a meal plan.*
RELEVANT • Is this goal connected to what you want to achieve**? • If yes, Why? • Are you capable of achieving it?	*Yes, it is definitely connected to what I want to achieve. I can do it!*

** If the goal is not relevant or connected to your desired outcome, don't attempt it now.

TIMELY • What timeframe is realistic?	*I want to achieve this within 4 weeks of starting the program.*

Your SMART Goal

The end goal could be:

"I want to reduce the time spent thinking about food daily. I will limit how long I think about preparing the current meal to a maximum of 10 minutes, accomplishing this within 4 weeks of starting the program. To achieve this, I'll utilise meal planning. When checking my progress, I'm not meeting the goal if I exceed 10 minutes of thoughts or planning for the immediate meal."

When you have your SMART goals, list them on the *Goal-o-meter* worksheet.

Key Questions to Ask Yourself

Apart from reviewing your set goals, there are additional ways to track your progress. Consider the specific points outlined at the start of this chapter, go through them, and reflect on how they apply to you. Concentrate on the crucial aspects that prompted you to embark on this program. Alternatively, you can use the following eight general questions. Establish a baseline for how you rate yourself regarding the goals or questions at the beginning of the program. Then, repeat every two weeks or whenever you wish to check in on your progress.

General questions about emotional eating:

- Do you seek comfort in food when you're feeling down, overwhelmed or stressed?
- Do you think about or eat food when you're happy or want to reward yourself?
- Do you use food as a nutritional energy source for your body?

- Have you reduced the daily amount of time that you spend thinking about or planning food?
- Are you coping with not having food available as a way to shield your emotions?
- Can you identify when you are feeling an emotion?
- Are you allowing yourself to feel emotions without avoiding or distracting yourself?
- Do you feel like you are managing your emotions without turning to food for help?

FoodFeelingsFreedom (3*F) quiz

This quiz combines essential questions with a rating scale, offering a straightforward method to gauge your progress in the program. Like the questions mentioned earlier, take the quiz at the beginning of the program and revisit it every two weeks or whenever you want to check in with yourself.

You will begin with a higher score and finish with a lower score. You may not start at the absolute highest score (24) and end at zero (0), but your score is individual to you. The decrease in the total score indicates progress in navigating the program components and towards better emotional management and a healthier relationship with food.

The quiz has been designed so that the score for each question will also go from higher to lower as you progress through the key points of the program.

If your total score remains the same or rises, it indicates that you need to dedicate some time to gauging your progress in the program. Perhaps you need to spend more time on a particular component or you need assistance working through some challenging areas.

FoodFeelingsFreedom (3*F) Quiz

Date:_____

For all questions, please select the appropriate response.

	In the past week:	No	Sometimes	Mostly	Always
1.	Do you seek comfort in food when you're feeling down, overwhelmed or stressed?				
2.	Do you think about or eat food when you're happy or want to reward yourself?				
3.	Do you use food as a nutritional energy source for your body?				
4.	Have you reduced the time you spend thinking about or planning snacks or meals?				
5.	Are you coping with your feelings without turning to food?				
6.	Can you identify your feelings and emotions?				
7.	Are you letting yourself experience emotions without avoiding them or distracting yourself?				
8.	Are you managing your emotions without help from a crutch?				

Score: _____

FoodFeelingsFreedom Quiz

Frequently Asked Questions:

Q. What happens if I decide to skip the Activity component?
A. You can skip the Activity component, as we talked about in Chapter 5. It's absolutely fine as long as you have support or can make adjustments to your food habits without needing a temporary crutch.

Q. I began the program successfully and saw some improvement, but I've hit a roadblock.
A. It might be a good idea to rethink why you started the program and if it's the best timing for you at the moment. If you're still enthusiastic about it but could use extra help, try connecting with a supportive online group or seek assistance from a health professional.

Q. I'm making progress, but stress sets me back.
A. It's great that you're in touch with your feelings. When you regress under stress, it's a sign that you could benefit from more work on handling that feeling and associated situation. Try to figure out what triggers it and any persisting feelings, and explore strategies to manage them. If it gets overwhelming, don't hesitate to contact a mental health professional for guidance.

Something to think about:

Think about some of your current goals and re-write them using the SMART goal approach.

How do you know if you're making progress with a task? Do you regularly check-in to see how you're going or wait until it's finally achieved, however long it takes?

8

What is Going Wrong, and What Can I Do About It?

Embarking on any journey comes with its share of challenges, and it's crucial to recognise that smooth sailing might not always be the norm. It's okay to face difficulties, but what's more important is knowing how to navigate them when they arise.

Instead of identifying every possible roadblock and providing solutions to get you back on track, the aim is to take a step back, look at the underlying problem, and see what area of the program is affected. If the same issue keeps occurring, look at the pattern of the problem or your behaviour.

This is how you can troubleshoot and overcome challenges that may be hindering your progress in the program.

1. Identify the issue
2. Does it fall under one of the areas listed below?
3. What can you do about it?
4. Seek assistance if needed.

Identify the issue

Think about what's not going as planned or seems to be causing a roadblock in your journey.

Does it fall under one of the areas listed below?

Consider if the issue fits under any of these areas: your personal motivations, other people or external influences, logistical challenges, following rules, understanding what is required, or practising habits.

What can you do about it?

Explore ways to address the problem and get things back on track, such as problem-solving. If you need help with this, there is a *How to problem-solve* worksheet in Chapter 12.

Seek assistance if needed

Determine whether you can work out your issue yourself or require external support to get back on track. This could apply to you if you have difficulty problem-solving. Don't hesitate to reach out for guidance or assistance from supportive friends, groups, or health professionals who can provide valuable insights and help you overcome obstacles.

Possible problem areas involve:

- People
- Logistics and resources
- Rules
- Understanding
- Practise, practise, practise

People

Related to you: What drives your desire for change? Knowing and understanding your motivations is key. Do you want to succeed?

Other people: Consider how others impact your journey. Are there supportive individuals cheering you on or doing the opposite? If you can't control how others are affecting what you want to achieve, what can you control?

Examples:

- After diving into the initial chapters of the book and feeling inspired to make positive changes for your health and well-being, you discovered that sticking to the program proved challenging. Despite initially thinking that the desire to enhance your health would be sufficient motivation, it turned out not to be the case.

- After chatting with your family and figuring out a meal plan that suited everyone, a family member switched their plans, disrupting all your carefully made arrangements for that two-week period.

Logistics and Resources

Preparation: Is your planning thorough and does it set the stage for success? Preparation for and during the beginning weeks is crucial.

Menu planning: Look back to Chapter 4 for guidance.

Activities: Look back to Chapter 5 for guidance.

Examples:

- On your plan, you intended to prepare a particular meal one evening but didn't factor in the time and effort it would take, especially after a full day at work.
- You had to postpone starting the program because you forgot about upcoming family commitments.
- You spend hours prepping meals in advance only to realise you don't have enough freezer space to store everything.
- You wanted to include swimming in your list of activities, but it wasn't practical or convenient as there wasn't a nearby pool.

Rules

Meal planning or Activities: Do you have issues with following the suggested rules?

Examples:

- You understand the rules of meal planning, but when dining out, you tend to let them slide and go for whatever you feel like at that moment.
- Your favourite series dropped the latest season of episodes, and you can't resist binge-watching them over a weekend.
- The rules seem a bit silly, and you don't see the point of following them.

Understanding

Clear understanding: Do you understand the requirements of the program and the reasons behind them?

Seeking support: Do you need help to get back on track?

Examples:
- You're totally fine with making a list of activities to use and can't wait to do them. However, when emotions hit, you find it challenging to turn to the activity list instead of reaching for food.

- You understand and agree with all the components of the program, but you're having trouble seeing how the different parts come together to help you shift how you approach and feel about food.
- You know what to do at the various stages, and you've figured out how to manage some challenges. But now, you're looking for additional support to stay on track.

Practise, Practise, Practise

Effort: Be open to putting in the effort needed for change. Changing a behaviour or thought process requires practice and dedication. It's essential to actively engage in the intended changes.

Realistic expectations: Understand that success and change are gradual processes, and that not having instantaneous results is normal.

Examples:

- You want to gain better control over your eating habits, and there are numerous advantages for you to focus on this over the next two months. However, fully committing to the effort required during this time is a bit challenging for you.
- You observe that the initial success you experienced in the early weeks of the program slows down and

hits a plateau when you dive into the mental tasks. There are moments when it feels like progress has halted, and it takes some extra effort to move forward through the mindset stages.

Frequently Asked Questions:

Q. It feels like there is a lot of effort required when I think about all the steps in the program.
A. Seeing the entire program laid out in front of you might make it seem a bit hectic. To make it more manageable and shift from feeling overwhelmed to being able to handle things and succeed, take it one step at a time. Don't move on to the next step until you feel at ease with the current one. It might take a bit longer, but in the long run, you'll achieve success compared to not giving it a try at all.

Q. I get the hang of the "doing" parts like meal planning and doing activities, but the "mind" tasks are a struggle.
A. Dealing with the mental side of things can be tricky for various reasons. If recognising and dealing with emotions is a fresh concept for you, diving into this aspect might feel like stepping into uncharted territory. Getting support from a friend, a group, or a health professional can make this part of the journey more manageable. A good place to start is to consciously practise identifying and describing what emotions you experience whenever you notice feeling something or being in a particular situation.

Q. I really want to change how I approach food for many reasons, but it feels like there is always something derailing my progress.

A. This is where you need to ask yourself why you're so keen on changing your behaviour. What is driving your motivation? Make sure it's something significant and truly important to you so that this program becomes your top priority.

If other reasons or situations start overshadowing your plans, it might mean your priority has shifted, or you could be unintentionally sabotaging your efforts. For instance, some people resist trying something new because, deep down, they're afraid of not succeeding. Another example of unintentional self-sabotage is wanting to reduce weight but not succeeding because, subconsciously, they might not want the attention of dressing stylishly or being "seen" and possibly receiving unwanted advances. If you suspect self-sabotage, it may be beneficial to speak with a health professional to help you figure out what is going on.

<u>Something to think about:</u>

- Think about the last time you had to troubleshoot a problem. How did you do it?

- If you're used to problem-solving, do you limit yourself to the first couple of ideas you think of or do you brainstorm and think broadly?

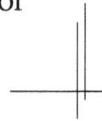

9

When to Stop…
and What's Next?

Exploring new things and seeing positive changes can be exciting, but figuring out when to stop can be tricky. While there's typically a suggested endpoint, what if you feel you're not quite ready to wrap it up? What if you want to keep going for a bit longer? This program is designed to conclude after eight weeks, allowing individuals to notice a positive shift in their thoughts and behaviours. However, you have the flexibility to extend beyond this timeframe if you're not ready to bring it to a close.

The Importance of Goals

By the time eight weeks roll around, you might have tried stepping away from the program or powering through each week. Regardless, you've been keeping tabs on how your thoughts and behaviours about food are changing. It all boils down to what you really want to achieve by going through this program. We've touched on this before in the previous chapters, but it's very important now. To reach your end goal, you need specific details. How will you know when you've hit that target? Your final goals are personal to you. While the processes might be similar for everyone, we all have our own concerns and issues. So, ensure that your end goal is 100% tailored to you.

In Week Zero, we introduce the idea of goals and what you aim to achieve. However, at the beginning, it's tough to figure out the ultimate possibilities. Typically, you begin by pinpointing the behaviours you want to stop or modify. As time passes, you start to grasp how your life could take a different turn, making you more brave in picturing what you want for yourself.

Trialling Off the Program

This program unfolds systematically over eight weeks, but feel free to hit the pause button and linger at any stage, especially once we dive into the mindset aspect from week four onward. At any time, you can stop following the individual program components or take a break from the entire program whenever you reach a comfortable and desired level of achievement. To gauge your progress, consider how you can tell if things are on track or if you're reverting to old habits. These signals are unique to you and tied to the reasons or emotions you've identified as triggers for turning to food.

For example, you might have realised that whenever you felt sad and needed a pick-me-up, you tended to reach for food in general or a particular go-to like chocolate biscuits. In this scenario, spotting yourself seeking out chocolate biscuits or any food when you're aiming for a feeling boost becomes a clear sign that you might be slipping back into old habits.

What's Next?

We're constantly pondering "what's next?" in everything we tackle; this program is no exception. What prompted you to think about and embark on this journey initially? Was it a personal choice, a step before considering bariatric surgery, or a precursor to engaging in a weight management program?

Regardless of the reason, your vision of "what's next?" is entirely your own. You might find satisfaction in your transformed relationship with food, your fresh perspective on engaging in enjoyable activities, or your newfound ability to embrace various emotions. Alternatively, you might choose to revisit and reinforce certain aspects of the program. It's all about what suits you best.

These steps will help you to know when to stop the program, and consider what's next:

- How your goals are progressing
- Trialling off the program
- Ongoing monitoring
- What's next?

How Your Goals are Progressing

Take a look at the goals you set during Week Zero or revised throughout the program. Once they're documented on the summary *Goal-o-meter* worksheet, it's easy to check if you're hovering around the >80% green zone. If your goals fall within that range, you can confidently say you've achieved or fulfilled them. If they haven't quite reached that zone yet, it's time to dig a bit deeper and keep going. What's hindering your progress? Is there a particular aspect of a goal that's causing a roadblock for the rest of it? If so, consider breaking it down and focusing on it separately. This exercise emphasises the importance of making your goals specific and relevant.

Do you struggle to figure out how to assess your goals? I mean, we're familiar with using numbers and scores from our school days, but when it comes to evaluating your progress on a personal goal, it can be tricky to grasp.

The following is another way to understand the *Goal-o-meter* scale.

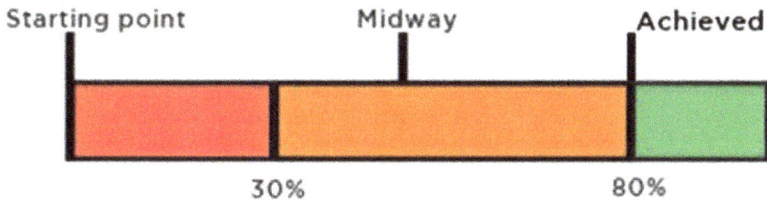

Goal-o-meter

- Don't be disheartened by starting in the Red Zone. As soon as you notice change occurring, you're out of there.
- At 30%, you hit the beginning of the Amber Zone. This is when you start to see positive changes happening as you work toward your specific goal.
- At the midway point, you'll see that you're making as much positive progress as you are continuing with old habits. After this stage, expect even more positive strides toward your specific goal.
- At 80%, you step into the Green Zone. At this stage, you're achieving or experiencing your goal most of the time. You're confident and doubt-free about reaching your goal. Being in the Green Zone is a solid indicator that you're on your way to ongoing positive progress toward your desired goal.

When and How to Trial Off the Program

Deciding when and how to ease off the program is entirely up to you. You can do it whenever you feel you're doing well and can continue without strictly following the prescribed content, rules, or pace of the program. This is a personal decision, and it's unique to each individual. Some are content to stick to the program, while others prefer to go through it at their own pace. There's no right or wrong way as long as you achieve your end result and achieve your goals.

The approach you take in trialling off depends on your current stage and what you're going through at that moment. If you're achieving what you set out for, you might choose to trial off close to completing the program. Remember, there are no strict rules saying you must go through the full eight weeks.

Ongoing Monitoring

It's suggested that you do a self-check every two weeks. While weekly check-ins are an option, the two-week interval provides a broader timeframe for you to observe any changes.

You can conduct your check-in using one or a combination of the following methods:

- Reviewing your goals on the *Goal-o-meter* worksheet
- Posing the Key Questions from Chapter 7 to yourself

- Asking your own specific key questions
- Taking the FoodFeelingsFreedom (3*F) Quiz

Initiate a baseline check-in during Week Zero and repeat at the end of weeks two, four, six, and eight. Feel free to adjust your progress based on how you're doing—whether it's pausing to focus on something specific or realising you're almost there and contemplating completing the program.

What's Next?

No matter what your "what's next?" entails, there might be some areas, whether related to food or emotions, that you need to keep practising. Since your old habits were deeply rooted, replacing them with new ones will take time and consistent effort. As you reintroduce certain behaviours, like rewarding yourself with food or drink, it's crucial to check in with yourself. Remind yourself that it's a conscious choice and you're in control. You recognise that you were mindful of the emotions tied to the activity or event, and you make a conscious choice to reward yourself in this way. The food or drink is secondary to acknowledging and experiencing whatever emotions were present at the time. Keep monitoring your progress toward your goals. If you find yourself slipping back into old ways, identify specific areas to focus on and set new goals to work towards. Embark on your next phase or program when you feel ready.

Frequently Asked Questions:

Q. Is it enough to be 'almost there' with my goals?
A. If being 'almost there' implies that you believe you've reached the Green Zone or are over 80% of the way there, then yes, you can consider trialling off or graduating from the program.

Q. Why, after finishing the program and going my own way, have I returned to my old habits after six weeks?
A. It's normal to find yourself reverting to old habits. Keep in mind, you've been practising those old habits for many years, so forming new ones in their place will require time and ongoing effort.

Q. Can I keep meal planning without the rule aspect if I've finished the program?
A. Absolutely. Meal planning is a valuable tool for various reasons and can be continued for as long as you find it beneficial.

<u>Something to think about:</u>

- When you start a program, do you see it through to the end, or see how you go and stop it when you feel you've achieved what you intended?

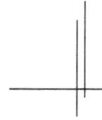

- What's next for you?

10

Bringing It All Together

You're approaching an end to all the information about understanding feelings and emotions and their connection to your eating habits. By now, you've done some self-reflection, possibly taken a quiz, and realised you're an emotional eater.

Which of the following can you put your hand up for?

- Your feelings and emotions, whether they're positive or negative, play a significant role in influencing your food choices.
- Are you facing challenges managing your weight? It's not just about losing weight but maintaining a comfortable and healthy balance.
- If you're trying to reduce weight, have you experienced successes only to be derailed by emotional situations

that send you spiralling back to square one? And, if you've been trying over your lifetime, have you turned the process of trying different diets into a hobby?

- Your emotional relationship with food has extended beyond yourself to others in your life: your children, partner, or someone else.
- When you need comfort or a reward, is food or drink your first choice?
- Despite attempts to create meal plans, emotional impulses often lead to unplanned purchases, derailing your plans.
- Even when you manage to plan a meal and buy the ingredients, unforeseen circumstances can disrupt your plans, resulting in either a cooking frenzy for future meals or discarding spoiled food.
- When dining out with friends, your menu choice depends on your current feelings or mood. Sometimes, the thought of what you could eat overshadows the joy of connecting with others.

All these challenges can be overcome by changing your relationship with food and learning to manage your feelings and emotions. Let me guide you along the path of *Food, Feelings and*, ultimately, *Freedom*.

Starting with the basics, the focus of the program is on becoming aware of your emotions, understanding the role of food in your life and identifying what needs to happen before changing any behaviour. Then, explore the three essential elements: Food, Activities and Mindset. Each is thoroughly examined, with the Food element focusing on adopting food as fuel, changing your perspective, and incorporating meal planning and the associated rules. The Activities element discusses the role of activities in transitioning, choosing activities for various reasons, and expanding your interests. The Mindset element guides you through understanding and managing your emotional mind, covering emotional awareness, identifying physical sensations, describing emotions, choosing to experience them, and gaining some control.

After delving into the content of each element, you'll be introduced to other program concepts, including monitoring progress, setting goals, self-monitoring, and regular check-ins. Learn troubleshooting techniques if things don't go as planned, focus on the process rather than specifics, and seek assistance if needed. The concepts conclude by reviewing your goal progress, ongoing monitoring and determining when you're ready to complete the program.

Here's how your life could change after completing the program:

- Your eating and drinking choices are now conscious decisions.
- You no longer label food as good or bad; judgments and value statements are gone. Food is seen more literally and is a necessary part of your body's energy requirements.

- Food loses its power over you; you decide what and when to consume.
- Informed food decisions are based on nutritional value and matching your needs with what's available.
- Repeatedly eating the same foods is acceptable and desired; novelty is no longer the main aim.
- You have control over food, which is integrated into your life.
- Emotionally, you are more self-aware, understanding triggers and managing uncomfortable feelings.
- Uncomfortable feelings and emotions are no longer feared, allowing you to pursue your dreams.
- You have more time in your day and are ready to take on the world.
- The emotional shackles that constrained you are gone; you have mental freedom.
- Increased confidence and pride in your achievements boost your self-worth.

For your convenience, visit the *www.FoodFeelingsFreedom.com.au* website. You can download and print all the worksheets and the full program. Complete the 3*F Quiz and explore links to online support groups and other program-related offers.

If you're ready, turn the page and take the next step towards your new life...

11

The 0+8 Week Program

The program's elements have been introduced in the previous chapters, and it's now time to combine them into an 8-week plan. If you still struggle with your relationship with food after eight weeks, you can continue the program for as long as necessary. If you find that your mindset about food is still stubborn, you can restart the program at week three.

You can complete this program on your own or with others in your household, although the other members don't have to follow the meal rules unless they share similar issues or desires. The meals are planned for two-week periods, allowing for some variety without feeling too restrictive. Having four breakfast options to choose from over two weeks feels better than being limited to just two options in a single week.

Week Zero

Food

Ask yourself the following questions to help you decide when to start and plan your meals for the first two weeks:

- Are you the only one following this meal plan, or do you need to consider others?
- Take a look at your upcoming schedule. Think about work, school, social events, travel, or any other commitments you have.
- Consider your time and energy for cooking. Identify when you'll have the time and motivation to prepare meals.
- If convenience is important to you, think about buying or freezing meals beforehand.
- Do you have enough storage space in your fridge or freezer to prepare meals in advance?

If you're not in charge of meal preparation for the household, think about which meals you can control to make them fit your plan.

Use the *Fortnight Meal Plan* to decide on meals and options for the next two weeks. Use this plan to make a shopping list or prepare what you need for the upcoming fortnight. When you're ready to start, fill out the *Weekly Meal Plan* for Week 1 and put it on your fridge, make it your phone's home screen, or keep it somewhere you can easily see and refer to it every day.

Goals

Consider why you're participating in this program and what you hope to accomplish. Keep your reasons in mind as you write at least one SMART goal. Your goal doesn't have to be perfect immediately, but it should include all the SMART aspects. You can review and improve your goals as you go through the next eight weeks. If you need help, you can use the *Goal-Setting* template provided.

Once you've established your goals, write them on the *Goal-o-meter* worksheet. You'll use this to track your progress throughout the program.

Emotional Eating Baseline

Before you begin, take the *3*F Quiz* to track your progress. This quiz will give you a starting rating score, which you can use to measure your progress throughout the program. Visit the program website to access the quiz.

Week 1

Food

Follow the meals and options you planned in the *Weekly Meal Plan*. To track how well you're managing the meal plan, use the *Food & Feelings Diary*. Note how you're feeling around meal and snack times. Did your food choices suit your day, or would you make changes in the future? Identify any speed bumps in the *Diary*.

Remember the rules!

Activity

Consider some activities you'd enjoy and start trying them out when you feel emotions surfacing and find yourself looking for food.

Mind

Begin recognising your feelings and emotions, particularly when you feel the urge to eat. Record them in the *Food & Feelings Diary*.

Week 2

Food

Follow the meals and options you planned in the *Weekly Meal Plan*. To track how well you're managing the meal plan, use the *Food & Feelings Diary*. Note how you're feeling around meal and snack times. Did your food choices suit your day, or would you make changes in the future? Identify any speed bumps in the *Diary*.

Meal planning for the next fortnight

Are you considering repeating the same menu for the upcoming two weeks? Review your notes from the last week and make any necessary changes. Begin planning the menu and preparation for the next fortnight, utilising the *Fortnight Meal Plan* to help you.

Remember the rules!

Activity

Utilise the *Activity list* to write down a variety of activities you could engage in. Remember to include at least four activities per reason, that serve specific purposes such as rewarding, comforting or another. Additionally, select a minimum of six activities for general use. Aim for a diverse range of activities to keep things interesting.

Remember the rules!

Mind

Continue recognising your feelings and emotions, particularly when you feel the urge to eat. Record them in the *Food & Feelings Diary*.

Emotional Eating Progress

It's time to assess your progress. You can either review your key questions or take the *3*F Quiz* on the program website. Don't feel disheartened if you don't see a change or drop in your 3*F score; it's still early in the program.

Week 3

Food

Follow the meals and options you planned in the *Weekly Meal Plan*. To track how well you're managing the meal plan, use the *Food & Feelings Diary*. Note how you're feeling around meal and snack times. Did your food choices suit your day, or would you make changes in the future? Identify any speed bumps in the *Diary*.

Remember the rules!

Activity

Feel free to expand the list of activities if you're seeking more variety or options.

Remember the rules!

Mind

Keep recognising and acknowledging your feelings and emotions, even those unrelated to food. Start a *ThinkFeelBody Connection* worksheet for each feeling that you recognise.

Over the weeks, you'll gradually complete all the components for each feeling.

Week 4

Food

Follow the meals and options you planned in the *Weekly Meal Plan*. To track how well you're managing the meal plan, use the *Food & Feelings Diary*. Note how you're feeling around meal and snack times. Did your food choices suit your day, or would you make changes in the future? Identify any speed bumps in the *Diary*.

Meal planning for the next fortnight

Are you considering repeating the same menu for the upcoming two weeks? Review your notes from the past weeks and make any necessary changes. Begin planning the menu and preparation for the next fortnight, utilising the *Fortnight meal plan* to help you.

Remember the rules! You can include one unplanned Flexible meal in Week 5.

Activity

Have you reviewed your list of activities? Do you need to add or remove any activities? What about extending your list to activities you would like to try?

Remember the rules!

Mind

This week, keep focusing on recognising how feelings and emotions affect your body. Some emotional body sensations might be easier to identify than others, so take your time learning about yourself. This activity will continue throughout the rest of the program as you encounter feelings and emotions. Refer to Chapter 6 again as needed.

Emotional Eating Progress

It's time to assess your progress. You can either review your key questions or take the *3*F Quiz* on the program website. This is the midway point of the program, so you will start to see a change or drop in your 3*F score. How are you feeling about your progress?

Goals

Do you need to revisit your initial SMART goal and consider setting more goals? Have you checked the progress of your initial goal on the *Goal-o-meter*? Is it in the Amber Zone yet?

Week 5

Food

Follow the meals and options you planned in the *Weekly Meal Plan*. To track how well you're managing the meal plan, use the *Food & Feelings Diary*. Note how you're feeling around meal and snack times. Did your food choices suit your day, or would you make changes in the future? Identify any speed bumps in the *Diary*.

Remember the rules! You can include one unplanned Flexible meal this week.

Activity

Feel free to expand the list of activities if you're seeking more variety or options.

Remember the rules!

Mind

This week, you'll be directly describing your feelings and emotions. Just like you've practised describing food without assigning value labels, now you'll do the same for how your emotions impact your mind and body. The challenge here is to refrain from automatically labelling the emotion as good or bad. Try to see the feeling for what it truly is without adding any value labels. Refer to Chapter 6 again as needed.

Continue completing the *ThinkFeelBody Connection* worksheet for each feeling that you recognise.

Week 6

Food

Follow the meals and options you planned in the *Weekly Meal Plan*. To track how well you're managing the meal plan, use the *Food & Feelings Diary*. Note how you're feeling around meal and snack times. Did your food choices suit your day, or would you make changes in the future? Identify any speed bumps in the *Diary*.

Meal planning for the next fortnight
Are you considering repeating the same menu for the upcoming two weeks? Review your notes from the past weeks and make any necessary changes. Begin planning the menu and preparation for the next fortnight, utilising the *Fortnight meal plan* to help you.

Remember the rules! You can include one unplanned Flexible meal this week.

Activity

Have you reviewed your list of activities? Do you need to add or remove any activities? How about some activities you used to enjoy but have forgotten about them?

Remember the rules!

Mind

This week focuses on adopting a curious mindset towards your feelings and emotions. It involves changing your perspective on how you welcome and experience them compared with your past habits, especially with feelings and emotions you may have disliked. Allow yourself to feel the emotions and observe the accompanying body sensations, thoughts, and instinctive reactions as if they are something new. Approach them with a sense of curiosity and investigation, exploring what they are and why they are happening. The aim of this exercise is not to make you enjoy unpleasant feelings. It's okay if you don't like them. The aim here is to realise that you can experience them without feeling they are too uncomfortable and something to avoid. Refer to Chapter 6 again as needed.

Continue completing the *ThinkFeelBody Connection* worksheet for each feeling that you recognise.

Emotional Eating Progress

It's time to assess your progress. You can either review your key questions or take the *3*F Quiz* on the program website. How are your answers or your 3*F score going? Can you see a noticeable change? How are you feeling about your progress?

Goals

Check the progress of your goals on the *Goal-o-meter*? Are they nearing the Green Zone yet?

Week 7

Food

Follow the meals and options you planned in the *Weekly Meal Plan*. To track how well you're managing the meal plan, use the *Food & Feelings Diary*. Note how you're feeling around meal and snack times.

Remember the rules! You can include two unplanned Flexible meals this week.

Activity

Feel free to expand the list of activities if you're seeking more variety or options.

You can start relaxing the rules for Activities now.

Mind

This week, the focus extends beyond feelings and emotions to changing your mindset. It's about viewing circumstances, situations, and everything else from a different or positive perspective. You can ask yourself, "Is there another way to look at this situation?" or "What advice would I give to a friend facing this issue?" The challenge lies in considering positive and constructive perspectives, rather than spiralling into negativity. Refer to Chapter 6 again if needed.

Have you completed the *ThinkFeelBody Connection* worksheet for each feeling you've experienced? If you have, what have you learned about yourself?

Week 8

Food
Follow the meals and options you planned in the *Weekly Meal Plan*.

Remember the rules! You can include two unplanned Flexible meals this week.

Activity
Keep doing activities if you enjoy them.

The Activity rules are relaxed now.

Mind
This week marks the culmination of everything you've learned and experienced throughout the program. You can now recognise and identify when you're experiencing feelings that evoke emotions and body sensations. You understand that you can objectively experience these feelings by being aware of them, describing them, and approaching them with curiosity. While you may not like or enjoy all feelings and their associated emotions, you know you can manage them and continue pursuing your goals. Additionally, you've

learned that you can change your perspective and see things from different angles, which helps you solve problems and avoid being trapped by negative thoughts.

Emotional Eating Progress

It's time to assess your progress. You can either review your key questions or take the *3*F Quiz* on the program website.

- How are your answers or your 3*F score going?
- Can you see a noticeable change?
- How are you feeling about your progress?

Goals

Check the progress of your goals on the *Goal-o-meter?* Are they in the Green Zone?

- If they are close to the Green Zone, what part of your goal hasn't been achieved yet?
- If you need more time, consider repeating the last two weeks.
- Do your goals need refining?

If you're in the Green Zone for all your goals, congratulations!

If you've achieved what you set out to achieve, well done. If you haven't got there yet, return to the stage at which you feel comfortable and keep going until you do.

Once you have achieved your goals, it's up to you what you do next… Whatever you do, I hope you take some of the skills you acquired during this program and continue to use them in your future life.

Week Zero

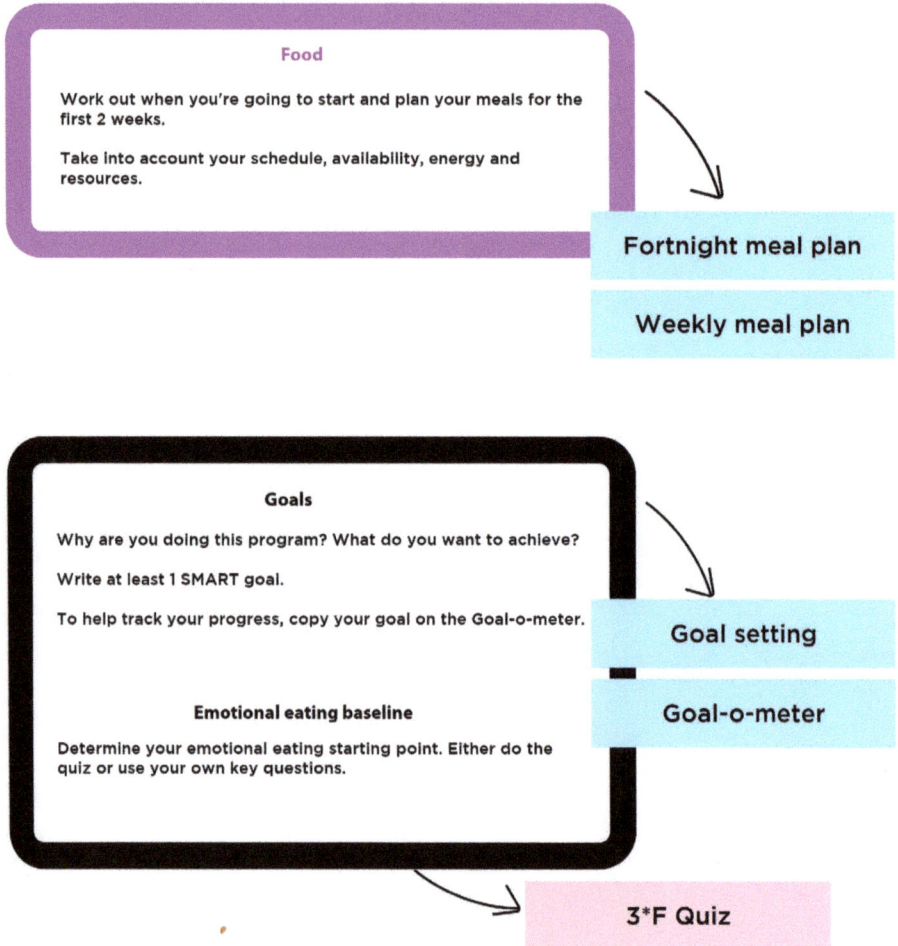

Food

Work out when you're going to start and plan your meals for the first 2 weeks.

Take into account your schedule, availability, energy and resources.

Fortnight meal plan

Weekly meal plan

Goals

Why are you doing this program? What do you want to achieve?

Write at least 1 SMART goal.

To help track your progress, copy your goal on the Goal-o-meter.

Goal setting

Goal-o-meter

Emotional eating baseline

Determine your emotional eating starting point. Either do the quiz or use your own key questions.

3*F Quiz

Week 1

Food

Follow the meals and options you planned.

Track how you're managing. Note how you're feeling, did your menu plan work, what changes would you make next time?

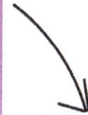

Weekly meal plan

Food & Feelings diary

Activity

What activities do you enjoy?

Start trying some of them when you feel emotional and looking for food.

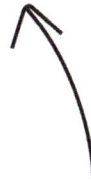

Mind

Begin recognising your feelings and emotions, particularly when you feel the urge to eat.

Remember the rules!

Week 2

Food
Follow the meals and options you planned.

Track how you're managing. Note how you're feeling, did your menu plan work, what changes would you make next time?

Meal planning
Review your notes from the last two weeks and make any necessary changes. Begin planning the menu and preparation for the next fortnight.

Take into account your schedule, availability, energy and resources.

Weekly meal plan

Food & Feelings diary

Fortnight meal plan

Activity

Write down a variety of activities
4+ activities per specific feeling
6+ activities for general use

Activity list

Mind

Continue recognising your feelings and emotions, particularly when you feel the urge to eat

Emotional eating progress
It's time to check on your progress, review your key questions or ...

3*F Quiz

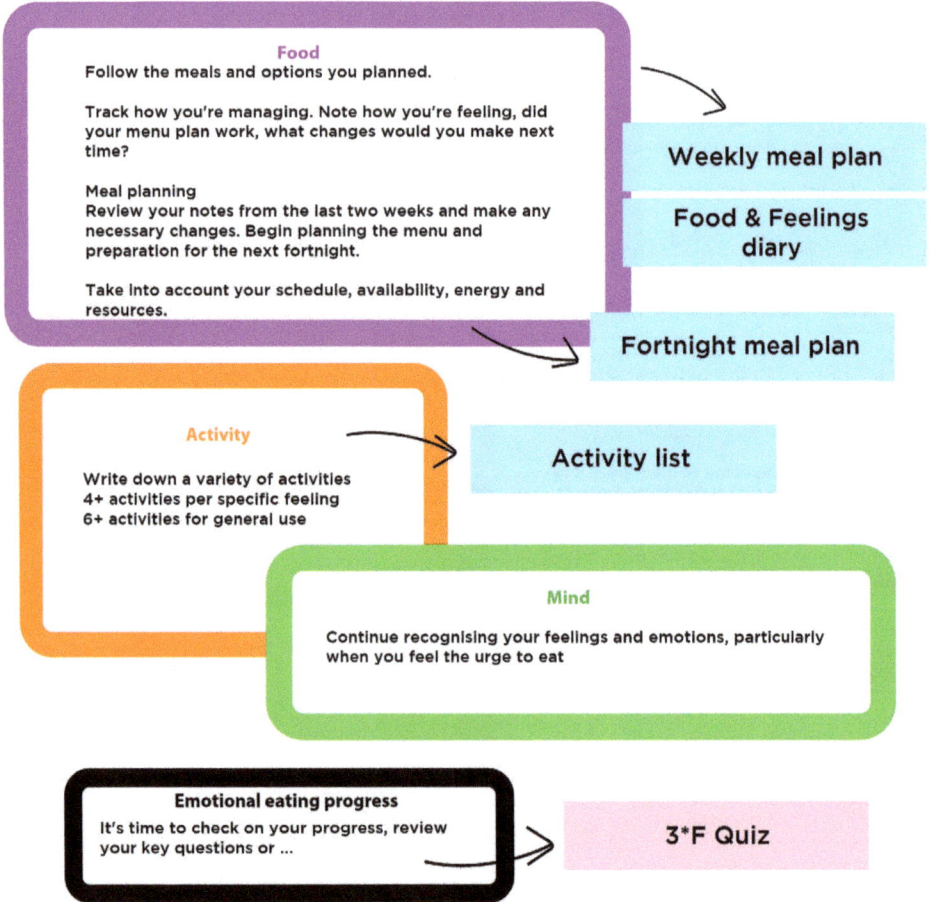

Remember the rules!

Week 3

Food

Follow the meals and options you planned

Track how you're managing. Note how you're feeling, did your menu plan work, what changes would you make next time?

Weekly meal plan

Food & Feelings diary

Activity

Expand the list of activities if you want more variety or options

Activity list

Mind

Keep recognising and acknowledging your feelings and emotions, even those unrelated to food.

Start completing a ˏ for each feeling you recognise.

ThinkFeelBody Connection

Remember the rules!

Week 4

Food

Follow the meals and options you planned.

Track how you're managing. Note how you're feeling, did your menu plan work? What changes would you make next time?

Meal planning
Review your notes from the last two weeks and make any necessary changes. Begin planning the menu and preparation for the next fortnight.
Take into account your schedule, availability, energy and resources.

☆ You can include one unplanned Flexible meal in week 5.

Weekly meal plan

Food & Feelings diary

Fortnight meal plan

Activity

Have you reviewed your list of activities?
Do you need to add or remove any?

Activity list

Mind

Focus on recognising how feelings and emotions affect your body.
Continue completing the ⟍ for each feeling that you recognise.

ThinkFeelBody Connection

Goal-o-meter

Goals Do you need to revisit your SMART Goal and think about setting new goals?
Have you checked your goal progress?

Goal setting

Emotional eating progress
It's time to check on your progress, review your key questions or the ...

Remember the rules!

3*F Quiz

Week 5

Food

Follow the meals and options you planned.

Track how you're managing. Note how you're feeling, did your menu plan work? What changes would you make next time?

☆ You can include one unplanned Flexible meal this week.

Weekly meal plan

Food & Feelings diary

Activity

Expand the list of activities if you want more variety or options

Activity list

Mind

Describe your feelings and emotions. See the feeling for what they are without adding any value labels to them.

Complete a for each feeling you recognise.

ThinkFeelBody Connection

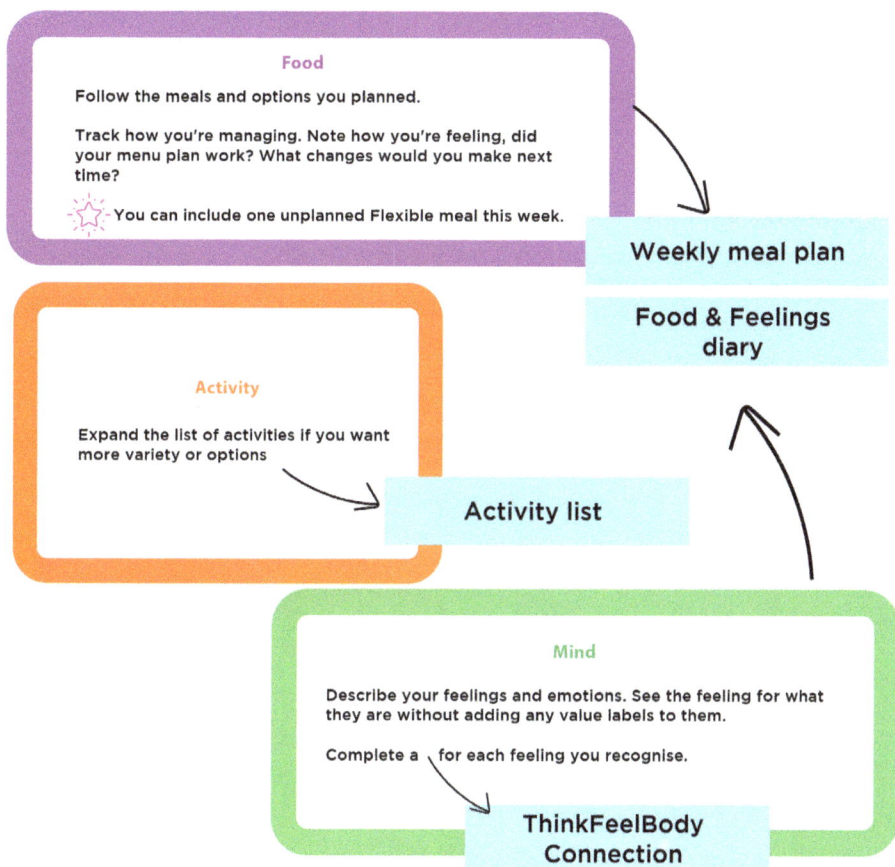

Remember the rules!

Week 6

Food
Follow the meals and options you planned.

Track how you're managing? Note how you're feeling, did your menu plan work, what changes would you make next time?

Meal planning
Review your notes from the last two weeks and make any necessary changes. Begin planning the menu and preparation for the next fortnight.

☆ You can include one unplanned Flexible meal this week.

Weekly meal plan

Food & Feelings diary

Fortnight meal plan

Activity

Have you reviewed your list of activities? Do you need to add or remove any?

Activity list

Mind

Adopt a curious mindset towards your feelings and emotions.

Complete a   for each feeling that you recognise.

ThinkFeelBody Connection

Goal-o-meter

Goals: Have you checked your goal progress?

Emotional eating progress

It's time to check on your progress, review your key questions or the ...

3*F Quiz

Remember the rules!

Week 7

Food

Follow the meals and options you planned.

Track how you're managing? Note how you're feeling, did your menu plan work? What changes would you make next time?

☆ You can include two unplanned Flexible meals this week.

Weekly meal plan

Food & Feelings diary

Activity

Expand the list of activities if you want more variety or options.

Activity list

Mind

Change your perspective and see things from a different point of view.

Complete the worksheet task. What have you learned about yourself?

ThinkFeelBody Connection

Remember the rules!

Week 8

Food

Follow the meals and options you planned.

☆ You can include two unplanned Flexible meals this week.

Weekly meal plan

Activity

Keep doing activities if you enjoy them.

The Activity rules are relaxed now.

Mind

Revise everything you've learnt and practised.
You can now:
- recognise and identify when you're experiencing feelings that evoke emotions and body sensations.
- understand that you can objectively experience these feelings by being aware of them,
- describe them, and approach them with curiosity.
- continue pursuing your goals.
- change your perspective and see things from different angles.

Goal-o-meter

Goals: Check the progress of your goals? Are they in the Green zone?

Emotional eating progress
It's time to assess your progress, review your key questions or the ...

3*F Quiz

It's up to you what you do next...

12

Worksheets etc.

To access and download all the Program resources, including the hidden worksheets and program, go to the Resources page on the *www.FoodFeelingsFreedom.com.au* website and use the password **RememberTheRules**

Fortnight Meal Plan

Flexible meal choices

Breakfast ☐ Lunch ☐ Dinner ☐
1.
2.
3.
4.

_____

_____

_____

_____

_____

Breakfast ☐ Lunch ☐ Dinner ☐
1.
2.
3.
4.

_____

_____

_____

_____

Snacks and Desserts
1.
2.
3.
4.

_____

_____

_____

Eating Out

Cafe/restaurant and menu choice
_____
_____
_____

Weekly Meal Plan

	Monday / /	Tuesday / /	Wednesday / /	Thursday / /	Friday / /
Breakfast					
Lunch					
Dinner					
Snacks					

Saturday / /	Sunday / /
Breakfast	Breakfast
Lunch	Lunch
Dinner	Dinner
Snacks	Snacks

Notes

_____
_____
_____
_____
_____
_____

Food & Feelings Diary

Day and Time	Place	Food/Drink	Was this on your plan?	Mood before	Mood after

Overall, my day was: (circle)

Activity List

_____ To reward myself

_____ _____

_____ _____

_____ _____

_____ _____

_____ When I am ...

_____ _____

_____ _____

_____ _____

_____ To comfort myself

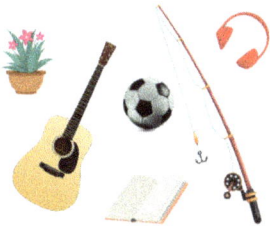

_____ _____

_____ _____

_____ _____

_____ Other ...

_____ _____

_____

_____

Activity Examples

Social Activities
Phone/Communicate with a friend
Visit a friend, family or neighbour
Go to the movies or the theatre
See your favourite local music band
Play with your children
Play with your pets
Invite friends over to watch a movie
Invite friends over to play Board Games
Invite yourself over to a friend's place
Go to an amusement park with friends

Things to do on your own
Write to a friend/family member
Play computer/console games
Write in a journal
Write a short story/poem
Play a musical instrument
Draw/paint/creative arts
Listen to some music
Knit/crochet/sew
Do a jigsaw puzzle
Do a paint by numbers
Read a book
Do some woodwork
Learn a language
Play a one-player card game
Look through your old photos/photo gallery
Browse social media
Learn something new on Youtube

Active things
Go for a walk/jog/run/cycle
Go roller skating
Go to the gym
Meets friends for a game of tennis/golf
Kick a ball around the park
Join Parkrun
Yoga/Pilates/Stretching
Run up and down stairs a few times
Go for a swim
Fly a kite
Go fishing

Things to do for yourself
Visit a spa for a massage/facial
Have a manicure/pedicure
Visit the hairdresser
Have a bubble/aromatic bath
Buy some colourful flowers
Try on some new clothes
Buy yourself a special gift
Sit outside and observe nature

What you can do away from your home
Visit and walk along the beach
Go to the movies
Go to a tourist attraction
Go shopping
Go to a festival/market/amusement park
Visit a museum
Go to the library
Watch a game of sport
Visit an animal sanctuary

What you can do at home
Do some gardening
Do some spring cleaning
Listen/dance to music
Do something creative/handiwork
Play with your pets
Watch television/stream a movie
Sit in/walk around the garden
Watch the wild life/listen to the birdlife
Admire nature

Goal Setting

SPECIFIC
- What do you want to achieve and WHY*?

*The WHY is important as it reinforces the reason behind your goal

MEASURABLE
- How are you measuring the success of the goal

ATTAINABLE
- How important is this to you
- Is this goal realistic

RELEVANT
- Is this goal connected to what you want to achieve**?
- If yes, Why?
- Are you capable of achieving it?

** If the goal is not relevant or connected to your desired outcome, don't attempt it now.

TIMELY
- What timeframe is realistic?

Your SMART Goal

Goal -o-meter

SMART Goal _____

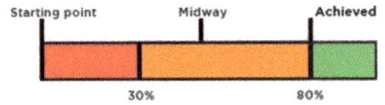

SMART Goal _____

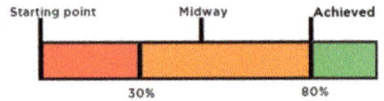

SMART Goal _____

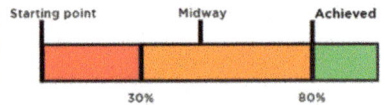

Think, Feel, Body Connection

When I'm feeling

_____

_____

_____

These are some of my thoughts

_____

_____

_____

_____

_____

_____

_____

_____

_____

_____

forehead

mouth

throat

breathing

heart rate

stomach

lower abdomen

hands

legs

* The idea is that you identify the emotion you feel, what thoughts you're having and where you feel body sensations

How to Problem solve

Consider the problem you want to solve as a whole or break it down in to smaller, manageable parts. This makes it less overwhelming to tackle.

What problem or part of a problem are to trying to solve?

1. Brainstorm all possible ideas that could solve it. Be creative and don't worry about finding the perfect solution yet. If you have more than 4 ideas, write them on another page

2. Pick the best 2 ideas. Take a closer look at each idea and choose the best 2 that seem the most doable and effective.

3. From the 2 finalists, which one is the winner? Consider all the Pros and Cons.

4. Put it into action. Try your chosen solution and pay attention if it works or not.

5. Keep observing. After seeing your solution in action. Has it solved your initial problem, how you wanted it to? If not, make some changes or try a different solution.

Remember the rules!

FOOD

1. Once you decide on your choices for the fortnight, you cannot change your mind

2. Decide when your Flexible meal will be. Is it in the morning, midday or evening?

3. The Flexible meal can be a different choice every day or you can repeat some meals throughout the two weeks if you want.

4. For the other meals of the day, you can choose a maximum of four (4) options for each of them

5. If you have morning or afternoon tea or supper, these are collectively called 'snacks', and you can choose a maximum of four (4) options.

6. If you eat out at a café or restaurant, order the same choice at each premises.

7. From week 5, allocate an unplanned Flexible meal once per week (optional)

8. From week 7, allocate two (2) unplanned Flexible meals once per week (optional)

ACTIVITY

1. Each activity can be done once or twice per week, maximum

2. Activities are time-limited.
- Doing any activity/hobby up to 30mins
- If the activity has a natural ending, then stop at that time
  - Watch one episode of a TV/streaming show, a maximum of 1 hour
  - Watch a complete movie
  - If you're reading a book, finish the current chapter close to the 30-minute time limit

3. From week 7, the Activity rules are relaxed (optional)

Afterword

As you journey towards understanding your emotions and making conscious food choices, I want to remind you to prioritise your mental well-being. While the strategies in this book can be helpful, they are not a replacement for specific professional advice.

If you're feeling anxious, have a persistent low mood, or are facing any other psychological challenges, it's important to talk to a healthcare professional. They can provide personalised support to suit your needs.

Remember, taking care of yourself means knowing when to ask for help. Your journey to Food, Feelings, and ultimately Freedom is unique, and I encourage you to reach out for support if you need it.

Best wishes,
G.G.Clement

Acknowledgements

I didn't write this book alone, not by a long shot. This journey has been a whirlwind of emotions and late-night writing sessions, made possible by the incredible support of some truly wonderful people.

Ann and my canine associate, Deeni, have been my partners in crime from day one and deserve a special shout-out. They've witnessed the evolution of this book, from multiple scattered notes to late-night typing marathons. My horizontal filing system was vast. At times, notes and notebooks were on multiple tables and in numerous rooms. I suspect they thought we wouldn't get to the end, but we have.

Let's not forget the crash test dummies of the written program structure—my dear neighbours and friends, Barry, Dorothy, Sue, Leanda, and Jo. You've bravely ventured into the uncharted waters of my ideas, offering feedback and encouragement along the way.

A huge round of applause to the unwavering support squad: Lisa, Mitchell, Nikki, Chris B, Praveen, Tony C, Thelma and the English family. Your encouragement and belief in this project kept me on track through the tough times.

Special thanks to my Alpha readers, Kate and Fabrina. Your insights and feedback saved my sanity and helped shape the complex thoughts swirling in my mind into coherent words on the page.

As we dive into the world of turning this program into an online course, Leisa has been a beacon of hope with her assistance. Here's to this and many more collaborations in the future.

Shout out to Kerrie (@kerriedoolan_artist), the genius behind the stunning cover image. With her incredible talent, Kerrie took my vision and brought it to life, creating a 3D structure that perfectly captured the essence of this book.

To all the neighbours, friends, and curious people who have shown interest in this project, thank you for joining me on this wild ride. Your enthusiasm and encouragement have meant the world to me.

Finally, to my mother, who shared an unwavering love and respect for books. I know you're no longer here, but we've achieved this together.

About the Author

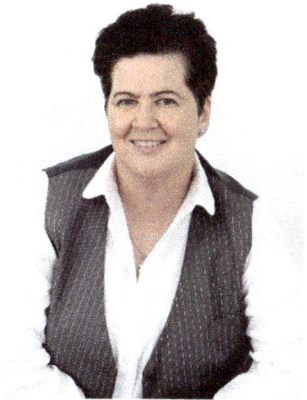

G.G. Clement is a passionate advocate for emotional well-being. With a background in nursing, midwifery, and psychology and over 25 years of clinical practice, she has gained extensive knowledge in the fields. She has delved into various psychological concepts and strategies that are the foundation of her book *Food, Feelings, and Freedom*. Her foremost belief is that everyone has the capacity for change, and her mission is to empower readers on this transformative journey.

In her free time, she is a lifelong student and enjoys being creative with almost anything. She is also a budding hobby orchardist and loves to take her dog for a walk. G.G. Clement resides in Queensland, Australia, and is always exploring new ways to promote emotional well-being and personal growth.

Notes

www.ingramcontent.com/pod-product-compliance
Lightning Source LLC
Chambersburg PA
CBHW052112030426
42335CB00025B/2955